ACUPUNCTURE:
A STRESS-BASED MODEL

Revised third edition

BY ROBERT HALE

Published by
AVICENNA
C/ R. Curtoys Gotarredona, 1, Esc. 2, 2B
07840 Santa Eulària des Riu
Spain

ISBN: 978-84-120109-5-4

Contents

CONTENTS

Interview with Hans Selye

The following is an excerpt from an interview with Hans Selye[1], who has been called the "father of Stress" owing to his ground-breaking research work in the mid-20th century.

Hans Selye: *'The whole concept arose from the observation that, in addition to specific diseases, such as a gastric ulcer or (unintelligible) or tuberculosis, there is a syndrome, a set of manifestations, a set of disease signs, which is common to all diseases, for example if you lose your appetite, you feel ill, you have no energy, you want to lie down rather than get up. And when I was a medical student I became very interested in it, and it seemed to me an obvious thing that should exist, that there should exist such a thing as what I called at the time the 'syndrome of just being sick', being sick from anything, and when I published my first paper on it, some ten years after I first confronted that problem as a medical student, I published it in the British journal Nature under the title, "A syndrome produced by various noxious agents".'*

Interviewer: *'What are the diseases of stress?'*

Hans Selye: *'Well you know, actually, stress plays a factor, plays a certain role in any disease because any disease causes an increased demand - you always have to come back to this definition in order to understand - but there are some diseases in which stress is a decisive factor, and there are a whole lot of diseases which have no apparent cause, the people have been looking for the cause of it for a long time but there is no cause, because the cause is just any effort, anything that causes stress.'*

1   Google. Selye. Youtube. Upload by drbrianpsych. n.d. Accessed May 28, 2022. https://www.youtube.com/watch?v=YJCeDtNh_Aw

Dedication to Dr. Gianfranco Miotto

Quite how young Gianfranco Miotto learned his acupuncture will never be known. He was an orphan and had been brought up in an institute. His schooling did not go beyond what was then compulsory (we are in Italy in the 1940s), but he was intelligent and an avid reader. He was also an engaging and charismatic young man, traits which took him a long way in many senses.

I was told that he began practising as a young man, treating the country people in the vicinity of his home, on their beds or kitchen tables. He evidently helped a lot of people, as he soon established a large practice, taking proper premises in the city of Treviso, north-eastern Italy. There he practised until, hounded by the medical establishment, he took his young family off to South America to begin a new life. In Paraguay he rose to the heights of society, with a busy practice in Asunción and counting the then President among his clients. Life in Paraguay treated him kindly until turns of events led to one of those episodes that occur from time to time, when a beleaguered dictator finds scapegoats for his country's troubles in the foreign population, and summarily expels them. Although he had been a favourite, Dr. Miotto was not immune from this, as intrigues within the presidential entourage had worked to sour his relations with those who mattered most. In the exodus he lost most of his wealth and belongings, and so, back in Italy once more, he had to start again almost from scratch.

I first met him, and was for a few years taught and mentored by him, several years after his return to Italy. I was, of course, also a patient, and he cured me rapidly and definitively of the hay fever that had badly tortured me every spring and early summer.

ACUPUNCTURE: A STRESS-BASED MODEL

Dr. Miotto's acupuncture was unorthodox. He had long discarded many of the traditional methods that he had studiously applied in his youth, learned from the few translations of acupuncture texts, both traditional and contemporary, that he could lay his hands on in those years. "Western people are different," he told me, "Trying to treat people adhering strictly to the traditional theories leads only to disappointment". He had worked with Korean émigrés in Asunción, and had picked up many ideas and methods from them. He was also an inventive man, devising many new techniques and constructing the devices necessary to carry them out. He believed in efficiency, effectiveness and ease of practice, rather than slavish adherence to tradition.

Dr. Miotto valued pulse diagnosis highly, but his interpretation of the radial pulses was not highly detailed in the sense that he was not interested in subtle nuances. His point of view was that there was nothing very precise to be usefully palpated, but basic perceptions such as of a strong or weak pulse, a hard or soft one, a deep or superficial one, were important indicators to him of how best to treat his patient.

Dr. Miotto had three favourite points: BL67, ST36 and LI4. The first because it is an effective point for any kind of pain anywhere in the body, and, as with most practitioners, many of his patients came with pain. The other two because he considered them psychosomatic points par excellence. I use the term psychosomatic as I believe he did, not to mean, necessarily, "somatic symptoms of psychological origin", but in the holistic sense of "disorders pertaining to the body-mind complex". Dr. Miotto rarely if ever saw a patient with any kind of condition for which he did not consider the psychological element to be an integral part. (Because of this interest he gained a doctoral degree in psychology from Padua University at the age of 45.) The first treatment of a patient would invariably employ these three points, to which he would add auricular points: *Shen Men* (on the right for a woman, the left for a man), and points corresponding to affected areas in the opposite ear to the side of the symptoms or disorder.

During subsequent treatments he would vary his choice of points. Along with one or two of the above three points, he would use one or two of a small range of other points, selected according to pulse diagnosis, most frequently LR3, SP6, BL61, KI7, KI1, PC6 or 7, HT7, SI3, GV20, CV4. Every two or three treatments he would revert to the scheme of BL67, ST36, LI4.

On the first and every second session thereafter he would also run down the entire length of the back from occiput to sacrum, on the GV and BL meridians, as well as up the arms from LI11 and across the upper trapezius region, with his mechanised equivalent of the plum blossom hammer. He had invented and produced an electrically operated contraption to make the task easier. Some patients liked it, some hated it. He saw this treatment as somehow priming the system to amplify the effect of his needles, as well as pressing the "reset" button of autonomic control.

Then there were his symptomatic techniques. Additional, local points were employed on top of the general protocol outlined above. For localised pain and trigger points he used a contactless mesotherapy pistol (now out of production due to safety concerns) to project small quantities of irritant (sterile saline) at high speed, sufficient to break the skin and form a small blister. For other locally manifest conditions he would select suitable local points, for instance, for hay fever, GV24, BL2, LI20. He invented a small probe to insert into the nostrils and deliver a small electric shock to specific points in the nasal mucosa. This was used for nasal hypersensitivity conditions like allergic rhinitis. Tendon inflammations would occasionally be made to bleed by pricking the overlying skin with a hypodermic needle followed by the application of a suction cup (typically, for ease, those with a manual pump rather than the traditional heated glass cups).

Dr. Miotto was a highly original, successful and respected practitioner. He never wrote anything (he was dyslexic) or taught formally. Although he was asked, he felt unable to teach "standard" traditional acupuncture, which he neither believed in nor practised. Yet I am inclined to believe that his acupuncture was the most traditional kind of all: one produced by a distillation of ancient concepts, his own empirical observations and reflections, tricks of the trade learned from various masters while "on the road", and his own ingenuity. Above all he understood people, and used that understanding in his clinical practice. That surely, is a more natural, real, and effective approach than sterile adherence to what has become today a stiff body of dogma.

In a way this book is a homage to Dr. Miotto, who was my mentor. The acupuncture that I use today derives from the observation that he got good results in a wide range of conditions by using variations on a very simple scheme. This reflects the fact that the body harnesses its self-healing potential according to a fundamentally simple scheme: the stress response. And from these two observations it is but a short step to the realisation that the basic mechanism of action of acupuncture is that of stimulating and/or supporting a stress response.

Preface

Legend has it that acupuncture was conceived as a treatment when physicians observed soldiers cured of various prior ailments after receiving arrow wounds in battle. I can relate to this. I often pick up scratches and gashes on my regular walks in the forest. I am of the opinion that these small wounds are health-giving, keeping the immune system primed and the stress response balanced. From simple observations such as this, at first applied in very simple ways, a method of treatment was developed, codified and progressively elaborated over many centuries into the complex system it is today. I happen to think that system is over-complex, heavily laden as it is with superfluous theory. I have always believed in keeping things simple, essential, and avoiding the temptation to micro-manage in the false belief that in complexity we are afforded more control. In fact, the contrary is true.

This is not a conventional acupuncture text. There are so many of those. Nor is it a manual of technique. It is a book of ideas and approach. I am aware that, as the ideas discussed are unorthodox, this book may provoke scorn and irritation in some traditionalists. I hope though that others will at least do it the justice of some reflection.

I studied Traditional Chinese Acupuncture in Italy under Dr. Ulderico Lanza, one of the first physicians to practise Chinese medicine in that country. I qualified in 1990 and was then mentored by my father-in-law, a highly experienced acupuncturist of some repute, who had taught himself acupuncture as a young man, but had then learned considerably more from the Korean doctors with whom he worked in South America.

Acupuncture is not an exact science. Each practitioner's own intellect and experience inform his or her *modus operandi*, to a far greater extent than is supposed to happen in our modern, so-called Evidence-Based Medicine. I am told that in rural China, each local acupuncturist has his own method, often passed down in the family over generations. For example, my father-in-law told me that on a trip to Hong Kong he learned, at a price in US dollars, the secret of success of a locally renowned Chinese acupuncturist. It was this: he only ever punctured the *Ting* points[2], and he sometimes punctured all of them. My father-in-law did not adopt this method: he developed his own, which was in continual evolution (but in which some things never changed), an evolution based on the outcome of constant trial and error and his own idiosyncratic style of inventiveness. Whether this kind of progress in medicine (trialling one's ideas on one's patients) is ethical or not, I shall leave for others to argue about.

I wrote this book because, in over twenty-five years of acupuncture practice, I have slowly but surely come to the conclusion that a lot of traditional theory is an unnecessary distraction from the therapeutic art and act. At best the mystique which surrounds it and its apparent technical complexity act as an elaborate piece of theatre (placebo!) for the patient. The codified traditional acupuncture most widely taught today evolved from a mixture of observation, trial and error, philosophy, reasoning, folklore, magic, tradition, and (despite its modern homogeneity) argument among rival historical schools of thought lasting many centuries. As such, it is unrealistic, in my view, to swallow it whole and uncritically.

Furthermore, I have not been able to ignore the fact that, since times of old, particularly in the East, there has been an esoteric convention in the teaching of any art: conceptual edifices were constructed in order not to facilitate the student's early access to the most essential knowledge, but indeed to prepare the student in other ways by hampering it. The reason for this was ostensibly so that the novice would not gain too much technical knowledge before acquiring the

---

2　Points situated, for the most part, at the ends of the fingers and toes.

wisdom to use it properly. Perhaps only a cynic (or a realist!) might suggest that it could also serve as an effective smokescreen to protect the master's status (only a true master could possibly understand such complexity), influence and income stream.

The former of these two reasons should not apply here. Anyone intending to apply any of the ideas presented in this book should already have professional-level knowledge of anatomy, physiology, pathology, clinical methods, patient care and management. They should also possess a knowledge of the general and locally specific risks of inserting acupuncture needles, and the necessary precautions attendant on this. Moreover, even though this simplified version of acupuncture will be immediately effective, the art will still take a lifetime to master.

With these considerations and my own clinical observations in mind, I have whittled down the theory underlying my practice of acupuncture to the minimum I have found necessary for effectiveness.

Let me begin here to set out my store. The principle messages in this book are:

- A good part of traditional theory, models and method is unnecessary embellishment, from the point of view of therapeutic effectiveness.

- The most important acupuncture effects are general and regional rather than specific to organs, systems, conditions or symptoms. Point specificity has been enormously exaggerated. All acupuncture affects overarching systemic control systems more than system-specific functions.

- Many of the effects of acupuncture can be seen in terms of a stress response, in the widest sense.

What do I think acupuncture actually does? Simply stated,

acupuncture captures the healing attention. A little more precisely stated, it engages the central nervous system in the production of a coordinated physiological response, which mobilises and directs resources in an effort to normalise physiological functions. To attempt to be more exact about it than this, one runs the risk of superfluous theorising[3] or dogmatising.

I wlll now engage in some fortune telling and answer in advance some of the main criticisms I envisage being levelled at this book.

1. It is arrogant to believe you can improve upon a centuries old art that has been developed by very intelligent people. I disagree. It might be seen as arrogance, but I prefer to see it in terms of looking beyond dogma, furthering insight and fulfilling my duty to my patients.

2. Reinventing the wheel is a pointless activity. It was developed by very intelligent people and it works just fine. I disagree. The first version of the wheel was likely to have used tree trunks as rollers for large slabs of rock. Clearly that could be improved upon. A cartwheel would be no good on a modern car. An ordinary car wheel would not do on a formula one racing car. In order to improve upon a wheel, one must understand its essential nature and the way it works. Nowadays that involves a sound knowledge of mathematics, physics and materials science. Conceptually, we need to take it apart and study how it works, and observe how each part contributes to its working, before building something better; for example, something simpler yet more efficient.

---

3   *Numquam ponenda est pluralitas sine necessitate* ("Plurality must never be posited without necessity"): William of Ockham (c. 1287-1347) in *Quaestiones et decisiones in quattuor libros Sententiarum Petri Lombardi* (Sentences of Peter Lombard). Otherwise stated as: "Don't needlessly multiply hypotheses". Occam's Razor (or Ockham's) is a heuristic that holds that among hypotheses, the best are those that rely on the fewest unverified assumptions, that is, the simplest.

3. Traditional acupuncture has grown organically over thousands of years. Therein lies its effectiveness. You cannot reduce its knowledge base without also reducing its effectiveness and scope. I understand this point of view. I am certain too that the scope of my system is narrower than that proposed by traditional acupuncture. However, I would be surprised if its actual effective scope were diminished. Traditional acupuncture has sometimes been considered a panacea for all kinds of diseases, but in my view that is wildly unrealistic.

4. This is a lazy person's acupuncture. I disagree. I am not a lazy person. It has taken me over 25 years of diligent, reflective practice to realise what I have written here. If anyone practises acupuncture lazily, he or she will obtain scant results by whatever system. Only by application, constant questioning, thought, and more application can we make any method our own to the degree where our results will excel.

5. There is no substance here, it is shallow. Well, sometimes the simplest things are in fact the deepest. In my other main discipline, osteopathy, I have never been a collector of techniques. A few techniques applied with the love and application of the craftsman according to the simplest of theoretical constructs produce consistently successful outcomes. The same is true with acupuncture. I have not been a collector of points and syndromes, but have appealed to the healing capacity of the organism with simple methods refined through experience, and hopefully applied with some healing craft.

6. This is a crude, blunderbuss approach. I would respond that it is not crude (simple does not mean artless - see above), but it is generalist. Treat globally to improve global health and

> specifics will most often right themselves.

> 7. What is proposed in this book is not acupuncture. Acupuncture means Traditional Chinese Acupuncture. I disagree. Acupuncture means inserting dry, filiform needles into the body for therapeutic effect[4]. Therefore, what I propose is acupuncture.

> 8. But it is not *real* acupuncture, by which we mean it is less worthy than traditional acupuncture. Well that is an irrational value judgement with which of course I disagree. Other than this, I can only reply to whoever might make this charge that I am pretty sure they do not know as much as they think they know.

I have not discarded all that is traditional, and for that I might draw just as fervent criticism from sceptics amongst readers. But I am above all pragmatic. If I have experienced what I sense to be the truth of things, I do not let any perceived lack of scientific plausibility stand against them. This applies particularly to diagnosis, including, to my own enduring wonder and intrigue, traditional pulse diagnosis. Traditional Chinese diagnosis is observational, and I have found the observed associations described by traditional texts to be insightful and rather accurate.

I do not attempt to cover all bases, simply to describe a method of practice which is simple and, in my experience, effective. I claim no absolute superiority for this method, only that it satisfies my felt need to achieve the most benefit with the smallest degree of complexity (a somewhat Zen idea, don't you think?). I feel this sincere search has been empowering to my practice because it has imbued the therapeutic act with added intent and potency.

---

4   Latin: *Acu* = Needle; *Pungere* = To pierce, to prick.

Preface to Third Edition

This revised third edition of *Acupuncture: A Stress-Based Model* contains a number of corrections and additions. On the one hand I had discovered a small number of inaccuracies in the first addition and on the other I have changed my mind about certain things. The additions concern relevant information from research, either new research or research about which I had hitherto been unaware. In particular I have added a new chapter on acupuncture point specificity, by which I mean the capacity for an acupuncture point to produce a range of distant or systemic effects that is distinct from those produced by other acupuncture points. I have also decided to greatly reduce the first chapter of previous editions (about stress), on the basis that the subject matter is likely already to be familiar to most readers. Further, the previous editions tried to be about both treating stress and presenting a paradigm in which acupuncture treatment in general is seen in terms of a stress response. Given the latter, the former now seems to me to be redundant. The other change in this edition is that I have sequenced and presented the material a little differently.

The general thrust of the book is unchanged. My contention is that acupuncture practice is overburdened by superfluous and questionable traditional theory. This book offers a simpler but, I believe, equally effective model for the practice of acupuncture. It bases this model on the concept of stress, rather than traditional theories such as *qi* and the five elements. An approach to treatment is proposed which does not rely on traditional maps of meridians or the traditionally described functions of acupuncture points.

Chapter 1: Observations and Propositions

'TCM' is not TCM (because it is not T)

The TCM[5] acupuncture taught in Chinese universities today is a standardised form established in the mid-20th century. John McDonald, author of *Acupuncture Point Dynamics*, explains:

The clinical experiences encapsulated in the historical literature of acupuncture are expressed consistently as point indications – this point is effective for this specific sign, symptom or disease.[6]

That is, point selection was based on empiricism and not on abstract theories.

McDonald continues:

The process of basing point selection on pattern differentiation, treatment principles and point "functions" or "actions" is a very recent framing of acupuncture created in the 1950s with the construction of "TCM".

In my estimation, this may well account for the apparent dissonance that exists between theory and pragmatism in modern acupuncture texts. On the one hand schemes and laws are presented by which one should select points to use, and on the other recipes of points for this or that condition.

I would also contend that truly traditional acupuncture would have varied considerably on the basis of the lineage of the practitioner, as in past times the healing art would have been passed down through families, and secondly, the spread of ideas and practices would have been extremely limited by today's standards due to geographic,

---

5   TCM: Traditional Chinese Medicine.

6   Post on social media on 1st September 2021 announcing the publication of *Acupuncture Point Dynamics*: McDonald J. *Acupuncture Point Dynamics*. Volumes 1 & 2. Self-published; 2020.

cultural and technological factors.

In reality, the so-called "traditional" acupuncture theory is a mixture of contrivance, guesswork and superstition in addition to practical empiricism.

It is irrational to swallow 'tradition' whole

It is irrational to swallow 'traditional' knowledge whole because:

1. People's minds are fallible, even those of very intelligent people, wise people, masters and authorities in their fields. Everybody has hidden biases, everybody is ignorant to some degree, everybody has a blind side, a stupid side, everybody makes untenable assumptions or overlooks relevant information.

2. In the East edifices were constructed to limit and hide knowledge, not to explain or clarify it. It was a common device used in esoteric practices to adopt conceptual barriers to obscure knowledge, ostensibly so that neophytes would not have access to knowledge that they were incapable of using intelligently, safely and competently; but possibly also (it would not be unheard of) to protect position, status and income. Aspects of the TCM taught today might well derive from such smokescreens.

3. Throughout the history of Chinese medicine, different masters, teachers and authors have had disagreements about their conflicting theories.

4. Traditional Chinese models are like God: they can neither be proved nor disproved. The rejoinder that "the proof is that they work" is not valid. Many things in the history of the world have 'worked' for reasons other than our erroneous theories about them, even if superficially their workings seemed somewhat consistent with those theories. The

examples are so numerous it would be superfluous to present any here. I'm sure the reader can think of some.

5. In TCM rough rules of thumb and half-truths have become dogma. For instance, five-element rules such as "if the son is weak, nourish/reinforce/tonify the mother", or the Japanese dogma that "disease always begins with an insufficiency". In both cases numerous examples can be brought up to demonstrate the inadequacy of these heuristics either to explain pathophysiology or to guide treatment. Again, it is so easy to think of these circumstances, that I'll leave it to the reader.

'TCM' models are neither very empirical nor very cohesive

'TCM' teaches that points be selected based on abstract models and premises. These are neither empirical nor properly cohesive. They derive from a mixture of philosophy, mythology, tradition, contrivance, superstition and guesswork, all of which provided pieces of the conceptual frameworks used to interpret observed phenomena. The process that must have taken place of fitting clinical observations into the traditional schemes would be very much like forcing oval objects into pentagonal holes.

TCM models and theories are not credible

Qi does not exist except as a concept. Meridians have not convincingly been shown to exist as discrete physical or functional entities. Any subjective evidence suggesting them is most likely a composite result of the workings of the nervous system, blood and lymph circulation. The system of correspondences and point functions is too neat to be true. TCM speaks in vague and ambiguous metaphors. And TCM teachings about physiology are millennia out of date.

There is no *qi*

Many of the entities/functions described by TCM are rough explanations for the effects of composite functions in the body. *Qi* is one example. *Qi* does not exist as any kind of energy or force. There are different classes of substance/energy described as kinds of *qi*, so let us take *Ying Qi* as an example, the *qi* that is supposed to circulate in the meridians. *Ying Qi* does not exist as a discrete entity. What is supposed to be *Ying Qi* is simply the composite action of the nervous system and the circulation.

Channels/Meridians have not been shown to exist

Let me rephrase that. Channels/Meridians have not *consistently and convincingly* been found to exist as *discrete physical or functional entities*. There may be some suggestive evidence, but not enough to sway the balance of probability in favour of their existence. Indeed I have my own anecdotes which might suggest them. However, I would argue that any manifestation of the meridian system is not the work of a *discrete physical or functional entity*.

Meridians are composites of real things

Meridians are as illusory as constellations of stars. There are no lines joining the stars (at least I haven't seen them) and nor are there lines joining acupuncture points. Meridians are not anatomical or functional entities, but artifacts of diverse, complex, overlapping neural and circulatory phenomena. Any effects that we attribute to energy flowing in meridians are composites of phenomena such as dermatomes, trigger point referral areas, axonal flow, blood and lymph circulation. Meridians are maps, not the terrain. As maps they may sometimes constitute useful rules of thumb, but no more.

You can squash an amoeba into a rigid little pentagonal hole but it will not be happy

Traditional Chinese medicine proposes that all things can be classified as belonging to one of five basic classes, known as "elements", "movements" or "phases". This is contrived, simplistic and unrealistic. You might be able to squash an amoeba into a rigid little pentagonal hole, or an elephant into a big one, but they will not be happy about it. Moreover, for any one case the five phase model can account for everything and its opposite at the same time, and acupuncturists take advantage of this... uhm... fluidity. For this reason the model is not credible.

Breaking News: Fire and Wind do not exist in the body

Some of the constructs of TCM are best regarded as metaphors. Fire and Wind are two examples; in many cases also Damp, Heat and Cold. Is this not *obvious*? Yet surreal as I find it, reading what other acupuncturists sometimes write about acupuncture, it seems that it does actually need to be stated. You see, the more one repeats something, the more one lives it, the more one comes to regard it as literal. If people really realised these were metaphors I would expect them to give greater indication of that realisation than by systematically parroting modes of speech that are hundreds or thousands of years out of date. So regard this as a gentle reminder to those who are under the impression that a stroke really is caused by "internal wind" or that essential *qi* is really housed in the kidney.

More Breaking News: The spleen doesn't govern transportation

It is nonsense for any Western trained health professional to say such things as "the spleen governs transportation and transformation". The argument that "Chinese Medicine theory uses the names of the organs in a different way to Western medicine" is certainly true, but as a justification it is inadequate. The ancient Chinese obviously knew what the spleen looked like, and they could touch one from a cadaver. It was near the stomach and the pancreas, so they wrongly assumed it had a role in digestion. It was full of blood so they assumed perhaps that energy passed from the digestive tract to the blood via the spleen.

For this reason they also attributed to it the function, "controls the blood". This is nearer the mark (the spleen does, in fact, filter out and and destroy old, malformed or damaged erythrocytes) but expressed as such it is too vague to be of much use. And to extrapolate that it had some role in ensuring the integrity of blood vessels is a step untoward (the spleen was supposed to prevent the blood from extravasating). My point is that the ancient Chinese were thinking along anatomical and physiological lines but their knowledge was not advanced enough to attribute correct or precise functions. Their ideas were developed long before people really knew what that fist-sized organ near the stomach was for. Their ideas often have a grain of truth, as any suitably vague statement does about anything. But thousands of years have passed and because of the Chinese veneration for tradition, they have become dogma in an age when they are no longer adequate explanations.

Enough breaking news. You get my drift.

The real-world application of TCM is subjective to the practitioner

Examples:

Different schools of acupuncture place different organ-functions at different pulse positions. They cannot all be right, at least, not if we are speaking objectively.

In examining a case, five different masters will make five different diagnoses and propose five different treatments. Afterwards, all will claim a good result.

Modern Chinese research into acupuncture is unreliable

Although it does occasionally happen, it is quite unusual to read a study of acupuncture published in China that has reported negative findings either in efficacy or in support for traditionally proposed constructs. It is just not credible that well-conducted studies could be so uniformly positive. Unfortunately this casts a cloud of suspicion on all Chinese studies. They simply cannot be trusted.

TCM theories of pathology are irrelevant to acupuncture practice

The ancient Chinese were supreme observers of symptomatology, and their categorisation of syndromes (patterns) is coherent and accurate in its way. Unfortunately, while fundamental for the practice of herbal medicine, in my view its relevance with regard to acupuncture is minimal and basic. Basic of the kind that moxibustion is indicated when cold is a feature of the pathology. For example, there is nothing an acupuncturist can do with needles *specifically* to disperse Wind or Moisture from the body, for the reason that whatever the practitioner might think they are doing, in reality the body's response to *any* acupuncture is general and normalising, not specific to a particular symptom, condition, pathology or biomarker.

Acupuncture relies on the study of informational connectivity in the body

Acupuncture relies on the study of informational connectivity in the body, functional relationships and anatomical ones. It is just that I contend that so far as functional relationships are concerned, TCM models are unrealistic and much of its theory superfluous.

Many of the points traditionally recommended for localised condition are local points

Many of the points recommended for this or that condition or symptom are in fact points local to it. All points have a local action. Most points on the trunk seem to have ascribed to them predominantly local actions.

Point specificity for distant points is illusory

The specificity of acupuncture points beyond their immediate environment is an illusion. There are some distant points which are used with a frequency greatly outweighing the others. These have a very wide range of traditionally described specific indications. These points are on the limbs below or at the elbows/knees. The areas below the elbows/knees are generally more sensitive than those on the trunk or those on the limbs above elbows/knees. These are likely to be the most effective points for any treatable non-local condition or symptom.

Inserting a needle through the skin and into the body's tissues causes a tiny area of damage. The brain registers this and sends resources to the area to initiate healing. But the effect of this is not only around the needle. Although the strongest effect is around the part needled, there is also an effect in the entire body, and especially in the quarter of the body needled. For example, if a needle is inserted into the right foot, it will trigger a healing response in the right foot, the right leg, the right abdomen, and the whole body in that order of strength.

The system of attaching functions to points is not credible. It is too perfect. For example, no, there are no Wood, Fire, Earth, Metal and Water points with effects on the treated (non-existent) meridian according to their own elemental correspondences. It is all too neat and tidy to be real.

I contend that acupuncture points have local, regional and systemic action but beyond that, their supposed specificity is largely illusory.

Tender points are often acupuncture points

Anybody who works manually with the body knows that points in muscles or tendons can become tender, and that the locations at which they become tender when over-stressed is fairly predictable. Some of these points have been described by workers in the West in various terms (myofascial trigger points, Jones' tender points, Chapman's reflex areas, etc.). In many cases their locations correspond to classically described acupuncture points.

Not all acupuncture points behave like tender points

Nevertheless, not all acupuncture points behave like tender points. The tender points noted above are found mainly in muscular or tendinous parts. For example, acupuncture points on the fingers do not typically become tender in the same way, although they may be tender if there is some local inflammatory pathology or ligamentous sprain.

Point tenderness is a prime indicator for acupuncture point selection

One of the oldest forms of treatment is to massage tender areas. One may well ask whether tenderness in part functions as the body's call for help: touch me here, yes, ah, that hurts but it feels good! I propose that points (whether classically described or not) become tender when the structure or system of which they are part or reflexly related to is over-stressed, and that treatment of tender points by acupuncture acts to reset that structure or system in ways that diminish the strain. As nothing in the body can change without affecting everything else in the body, this treatment has both local and systemic effects. I propose that point tenderness is a most important indicator for point selection for acupuncture needling.

Points on the same facets of the extremities tend to have similar traditionally described indications

For example, those on the medial foot, leg and thigh all treat disorders of pelvic organs, whether they are classified as Kidney, Spleen or Liver points. Those of the anterior hand, forearm and arm treat disorders of the heart and chest, whether they are Lung, Pericardium or Heart points.

Points on the legs have more indications below the diaphragm, those on the arms more above the diaphragm

A very simple observation, for which no further explanation seems necessary.

The word is information, not energy

According to traditional Chinese medicine, acupuncture influences the flow of energy along the channels. As I mentioned above, I do not believe that any kind of *qi* exists as a discrete entity. Personally, instead of energy flow, I like to think of information flow and provision of resources. Instead of energy channels, I think of the nervous system and circulation. A needle inserted through the skin is a signal to the central nervous system to mobilise resources for healing to take place. These resources include blood flow, biological chemicals, the immune system, and yes, also the physical energy required for their mobilisation and use.

The response to acupuncture is a stress response

This observation, hiding here in the midst of all the others, is the main thing! Upon which all the rest is based. Acupuncture provides a controlled source of acute stress and as a consequence a mini *alarm* response from the organism. There is, in Hans Selye's terms, a local adaptation of physiology, and in many cases hopefully a general adaptation. These are temporary adaptations whose function is to reset homeostasis nearer to normal. As this is the main thing, let me shout it louder so that you remember I said it:

The response to acupuncture is a stress response.

We cannot micromanage physiology

The body cannot be micromanaged. What we have to do is to work out how to influence its homeostasis at a very general level, by means of stimulating the peripheral nervous system.

There is no tonification or dispersion, only normalisation

This observation follows from the previous two observations, and I am speaking of the longer term. In a patient with energy and resources that are not extremely depleted, *any* kind of needle stimulation within an normal therapeutic intensity range will result in normalisation. If stimulation is strong, it may provoke a short-term increase in expenditure of physiological resources and a local dispersion of energy (kinetic from blood flow, heat from the opening of the peripheral circulation), and this may be a useful thing in some acute cases. But after anything from a few hours to a few days local and systemic physiological parameters will tend to normal equilibrium, often at a better homeostatic setting than before. You may think you have "tonified" but if the body really needed to put the brake on, that is what it will do. And vice versa. Thus "tonification" and "dispersal" modes of needle manipulation are relevant only to acute pathology.

The main variables which decide needling intensity are our patient's constitution and energy level

Again I speak of treating chronic conditions. Given that all treatment ultimately has a normalising effect (not a specifically tonifying or dispersing effect) *except when the patient is severely depleted* the main variable which decides needling intensity is our patient's energy level. A very weak patient needs subtle stimulation, while some patients who are highly energetic or constitutionally hardy may not respond unless stimulation is strong.

If you stub your toe, your whole body changes

Any stimulus above a certain threshold affects the whole of the body through psychoneuro-endocrino-immunological changes. This may be temporary, but experience shows that repeated stimulation has a longer-term modelling effect on physiology. One might say such adaptation is a kind of induced allostasis.

An inner/outer and superior/inferior topographical relationship can be exploited

The medial surface of the lower extremity and the ventral surface of the upper extremity relate to the front of the body and the internal organs.

The lateral surface of the lower extremity and the dorsal surface of the upper extremity relate to the back of the body and the spine.

The upper extremity relates to the parts or the body above the diaphragm.

The lower extremity relates to the parts or the body below the diaphragm.

Potency

However, all points have a systemic effect and certain points seem to have a greater potency to effect changes that reach all parts of the body, regardless of the topographical relationships expressed above. I will call these points major points or *super points*.

A vertical / horizontal grid system can be used as a lens

Zhang Xinshu's Wrist and ankle acupuncture uses a zonal system to determine where to needle[7]. I find its delineation rather too well defined and rigid, but the notion is sound. To the vertical zones, in addition, I would add horizontal ones defined segmentally (dermatomes and myotomes) to focus the effect. Together the vertical and horizontal zones form a grid system which acts as a kind of therapeutic lens.

Gathering and focusing the healing attention

Needling constitutes a minor assault which gathers the healing attention of the CNS. Our grid system focuses it like a lens.

---

7   Xinshu Z. Wrist and Ankle Acupuncture Therapy. *JCM*. 1991;7:5-14.

Pulse taking is divining / dowsing

Different traditions and different historical times have used different pulse positions in different ways. Yet everybody has claimed that pulse-taking has materially and successfully aided their diagnoses. Let us perhaps naively take this all as being true. If that were the case, we would be obliged to concede that pulse taking is both reliable and subjective. This seems paradoxical. The only conclusion could be that it is akin to divining, like dowsing for water. Strange as this may seem to the reader given what I have written so far, I believe in divining. I believe in it more than I believe that e.g. the deep *chi* (foot or proximal) radial pulse position on the left wrist objectively reflects the health of our kidneys or the temporal characteristics of our kidney *qi*.

You are irrational even if you don't think so

You may have read the above statements and had an emotional reaction to some or all of them. I would be willing to bet that a not insignificant proportion of the people reading it will have felt annoyance, anger even. If that is you, I ask you to take ten slow, deep breaths then read it again slowly and calmly. Put a brake on the automatic inclination to think of counter-arguments. Throw your biases out of the window just for now; you can go, for your comfort, and retrieve them later on. Try, without them, to consider each point from a position of detachment, casting your unfiltered attention wide for all available evidence, and assessing it from different perspectives.

You are superstitious even if you don't think so

People tend to continue to do things the way they have always done them, not always because they are necessary, but because of the fear that they might be, and so leaving them out or changing them might make the endeavour unsuccessful or less effective. I know this because I do it myself. I am still weaning myself off it, a little at a time. If there has to be esoteric ritual (which of course can help), I want it to comprise essential, efficient, effective, incisive action. Effective in more than just a placebo kind of way. No bloat, nothing superfluous. Dumping superstition is part of this.

Chapter 2: Homeostasis, Adaptation, Allostasis, Stress

Readers will already be familiar with the notions introduced in this chapter. However, I need to review them, not least for my own benefit in developing my argument.

2.1 Homeostatis, Adaptation, Allostasis

Briefly:

Homeostasis is the rapid-response maintenance by the organism of physiological variables within ranges compatible with health.

Adaptation to longer-term demands placed upon the organism may require a shift in homeostatic norms.

This kind of shift is termed **allostasis.** For example, chronic **stress** requires long-term changes in the organism's neuroendocrine responses.

Allostatic load is a term used to describe the accumulated damage done to the body by repeated or chronic stress. This seems to me to be a misnomer. Load is load, impact is impact. The meaning is allostatic impact.

2.2 Stress

Hans Selye (1936)

In 1936 Hans Selye published his seminal paper on the physiological stress response[8], "a non-specific response of the body to any demand

---

8   Selye H. A Syndrome produced by Diverse Nocuous Agents. *Nature.* 1936;138:32. https://doi.org/10.1038/138032a0.

for change". By exposing rats to an array of unpleasant or damaging agents, he observed the evolution of the pathological changes in their bodies. Further, he categorised them into three stages which would occur in sequence if exposure to the the harmful agents was not terminated. This triphasic response was later termed by Selye the General Adaptation Syndrome. Selye gave the name of stressor to any stimulus resulting in stress.

It is of note that Selye was concerned with physiological responses. But of course, stress is also a mental phenomenon. Here is one description of stress taken from the work of a psychologist who has been prominent in the field, R. S. Lazarus[9]:

"Stress arises when individuals perceive that they cannot adequately cope with the demands being made on them or with threats to their well-being."

While Carver and Connor-Smith (2010) described stress as "the experience of anticipating or encountering adversity in one's goal-related efforts" [10].

Demands

Stress involves an interplay between demands and our perceptions, interpretations, feelings and behaviour towards those demands.

A demand is any event or situation to which a living organism must in some way respond or adapt. In place of "demands", we could just as well use the word "challenges".

---

9   Lazarus RS. *Psychological stress and the coping process*. McGraw-Hill; 1966. Lazarus and his co-worker S. Folkman later developed the Transactional Model of Stress. They described stress as "...an imbalance between the demands imposed on the organism, and the capacity of the organism to cope with those demands." (Lazarus RS, Folkman S. *Stress, Appraisal, and Coping*. Springer; 1984.)

10 Carver CS, Connor-Smith J. Personality and coping. *Annu Rev Psychol*. 2010;61:679-704. doi:10.1146/annurev.psych.093008.100352

Physiological, psychological and behavioural responses to demands have the aim of bringing about a satisfactory outcome. This may mean a return to the status quo, an improvement in one's situation, or even "least bad" damage limitation.

Demands can strengthen or weaken the organism depending on the nature, intensity and duration of the demand and the prior state of the organism. Beneficial stress has been called *eustress*. The usual term for damaging stress is *negative stress*.

Demands may be physiological, as in the above example, emotional, social, from our physical environment (e.g. climate, chemical pollution, ionising radiation), or biological (e.g. pathogenic micro-organisms and other parasites).

A demand can also be the insertion through the skin of an acupuncture needle.

Resources

The things that enable our capacity to meet demands we call resources. Insufficient, inadequate, or poorly utilised resources will compromise our capacity adequately to meet demands. Speaking in general terms coping resources include a variety of physical, cognitive, emotional, behavioural, social, practical, material and spiritual assets. Confining ourselves to a discussion pertinent to acupuncture being framed *as a demand*, our resources are physiological and psychological. It is not an absurdity to say that the healthier a person is in body and mind the better they will respond to acupuncture.

Acute Responses

Acute stress involves short-lived, relatively intense responses to recent events. In general they are normal and physiological, not pathological, that is, they are not "a problem" because they serve a purpose. During these reactions, increased sympathetic activity and adrenal medullary secretions stimulate certain bodily processes and inhibit others:

- The heart rate and force of contraction increase, and the arterioles constrict, increasing blood pressure.

- The bronchi dilate.

- Gastrointestinal motility and secretion are reduced.

- Sweating is increased.

- Glycogen is broken down into glucose.

These adaptations prime us for emergency situations. Emergency situations have been called "fight or flight" situations[11]. The urge physically to show aggression or to escape when faced with a challenge are primitive urges in all higher animals. While humans have the cognitive ability voluntarily to override these urges, the involuntary processes of our bodies still respond to them.

Although acute stress responses are generally functional, there are occasions in which there is a mismatch between the response and the situation. A response should be proportionate, neither a damp squib nor a wild over-reaction. Disproportionate responses may be problematic in various ways and to that extent we may call them dysfunctional.

Excessively intense responses may occur if a person has become over-sensitive to threat ("once bitten, twice shy"), either a specific kind of threat or through generalisation to all potential threats. Sensitisation of this kind can have survival value. If you are once

---

11 The "fight or flight" response has also sometimes been called "fight, flight or freeze" because "freezing" i.e. suspension of thought and activity, is one response to critical situations. However, it is important to remember that "fight" or "flight" would be adaptive (e.g. life-saving) more often than "freezing", unless of course, one is a possum.

bitten by a snake you would do very well to be wary of snakes in general. Not so dogs, in general. To be generally wary of snakes, if we are not a poisonous reptile expert, is sensible. But to be petrified of all dogs is unreasonable, as well as being disabling, as we will often encounter pet dogs. So the appropriateness of such conditioned responses is context-dependent. Sometimes people do become unrealistically sensitive and intensely responsive to mild threats which most people would say should not merit such a reaction.

It requires only a little thought to see how the above observations are relevant to acupuncture treatment. Inter-subject variability in reactiveness to acupuncture needling is a common observation, and will influence how we needle.

Chronic Adaptations

Chronic stress, on the other hand, involves adaptive responses to ongoing situations which are not going away soon. Typical situations of this kind are an unhappy marriage, mobbing or bullying at work, and debts or other long-term economic pressures.

The bodily adaptations required in these situations differ from those needed in sudden emergencies. When the organism is under constant pressure to perform or to meet extra demands, it requires a constant supply of fuel for energy production, and it needs a means of up-regulating its general responsiveness. The activation of bodily processes that occurs in acute stress favours the rapid but relatively inefficient breakdown of muscle and liver glycogen into glucose. However, long-term and constant challenge requires longer-lasting, more constant, more efficient energy production. Then, fat stores and muscle tissue have to be broken down to produce fatty acids and glucose for fuel, calcium is taken from bone to serve in metabolic reactions, and sodium is retained in the body to increase blood volume and maintain increased blood pressure. These changes are brought about under neuroendocrine control, especially by increased secretion of cortisol from the adrenal cortex and a general up-regulation of the baseline tone of the sympathetic nervous system (SNS).

A long-term situation of stress implies that we must always be on at least amber alert. Therefore to cope with chronic stress the general responsiveness of the body must be up-regulated, so we can respond quickly to the problems we expect to meet. This is like turning up the thermostat in your home. As noted, we use the term allostasis to talk about such longer-term physiological adaptations, in contrast to homoeostasis, for short-term righting responses.

Chronic stress responses are still generally functional (that is, appropriately adaptive to the situation), but they are a "Plan B". Plan A was to resolve the situation quickly. If this cannot be done, we resort to Plan B. Plan B is not as satisfactory as Plan A: it is a "least worse" strategy involving bodily changes which in the long term are quite costly in terms of energy and wear and tear *(allostatic load)*. The organism under chronic stress can be compared to a car engine running on an over-fine fuel mix: we have to use more throttle to achieve the same power, the engine overheats, and its components wear out sooner.

It is pertinent to point out that so far as physiological stress responses are concerned, the body makes no distinction between physical and emotional sources of stress.

The General Adaptation Syndrome

In his ground-breaking 1936 paper[12], Hans Selye described a set of general physiological responses to stressful stimuli, a pattern of responses that he would call the General Adaptation Syndrome.

---

12 Selye H. A Syndrome produced by Diverse Nocuous Agents. *Nature.* 1936;138:32. https://doi.org/10.1038/138032a0.

HOMEOSTASIS, ADAPTATION, ALLOSTASIS, STRESS

The General Adaptation Syndrome (GAS) proposes three "stages" of physiological stress, as outlined below.

- Stage 1: "Alarm": Response to a short-lived stess. Short-term bodily changes.

- Stage 2: "Resistance": Adaptation to long-term demands. Prolonged bodily changes.

- Stage 3: "Exhaustion": The body's adaptive capacity is exceeded due to exhaustion of resources and wear and tear.

In the light of the preceding paragraphs we can see that what Selye was describing are our responses to acute (stage 1) and chronic (stages 2 and 3) stress.

The term "stage" may lead to the misconception that they proceed in linear and uninterrupted fashion, and that stages 2 and 3 are inevitable results of the previous stages. But this is so only if a steady state of considerable stress never lets up. However, it is a common thing for people to be under chronic stress but to experience periods of heightened stress over and above that baseline. In that case their bodies and minds are "resisting" the ongoing situation but during short periods of heightened stress they produce "alarm" responses. They are not hopping from one "stage" to another, but they are displaying different and overlaid modes of response at different times, according to the circumstances. Further, if a challenging situation is quickly resolved, there will be no need for "resistance". Similarly, exhaustion is not an inevitable result of chronic stress, because life circumstances may change, eliminating the stress, or our abilities to deal with stress may improve. However, there is little doubt that unresolved chronic stress increases morbidity and shortens life. The exhaustion phase, if there is no recuperation, results in serious illness and/or early death either from illness or generally accelerated ageing.

But for the reasons stated, in later chapters of this book I will refer to *modes* rather than *stages* of the GAS.

Stress as a Common Denominator of Disease

It is almost universally accepted knowledge today that (excepting the relatively few conditions that are overwhelmingly determined by the genes) ill health, both acute and chronic, is a product of the interaction between our innate constitution and our environment, considered in the broadest sense. The latter includes everything around us which affects us - the physical, the biological and the social - in any way, from the time we are conceived onwards. All these things that impinge upon us, and produce some kind of response from us, may be considered potential stressors.

It follows from this that stress of some kind has a role in most ill health. For this reason I accept Selye's proposal[13] that it is a common denominator of disease. Further, and importantly, in contrast to our innate constitution it is an aspect of health which is amenable to intervention. I would go further: all methods of treatment which are effective and not suppressive of the organism's self-correcting efforts work on this basis, whether or not that is acknowledged. This includes, of course, acupuncture.

2.3 What Has All This Got to Do with Acupuncture?

First, stress is a common denominator of disease.

Second, acupuncture is a controlled stressor.

Third, acupuncture is adaptogenic: it modulates the stress response.

Put simply, most ill health will benefit from a reduction in the sum total of demands on the organism ad/or the improvement in the

---

13   See the transcript of an interview with Hans Selye on page vii above.

capacity of the organism to respond efficiently and effectively to those demands. So how can we reduce the load with acupuncture?

Well, we do, and I can envisage various rationales or general explanations.

1. We can appeal to traditional theory, "five element" theory for example, or theories about functional classes of points. Controversially, I state here my belief that benefits achieved through the application of traditional theory are illusory. That is, I believe in the benefits, but I do not believe that traditional theory has a great deal to do with those benefits from a technical point of view. It has a lot to do with them from another point of view. The practitioner has invested much, in terms of identification, in the system in which she believes she is intervening. This buttresses her belief and affords her confidence, a commodity (a valuable resource) she transmits to her patient, thus creating a context for healing.

2. At a simpler but more realistic level, we can employ points which have been found empirically to benefit a wide range of different symptoms, organs and systems. These are the points which are most likely to improve the organism's stress response in a general sense. They are adaptogenic points. Acupuncture may exert a generic, overarching, adaptogenic effect on neuroendocrine control. This, in my opinion, is a plausible mechanistic explanation for benefits mistakenly attributed to the specific effects of needling according to traditional models.

3. We can enhance the placebo. Many patients find treatment relaxing and pleasant, especially if an effort has been made to make the treatment environment conducive to relaxation. Relaxation facilitates healing, and can be a catalyst for a self-healing cascade. This may be a very different scenario

to that of hospital practice in China, but we should consider that an advantage, not a point of weakness.

4. We can exploit conditioning. Many years ago I noted patients' comments that, remembering the therapeutic context and act (needling) during their daily lives, they re-experienced the same sense of relaxation that they had during treatment. It is an ancient Chinese adage, I have heard, that "relaxation is who you are". Is it not true that healing is a form of getting back to our true selves? Since then, I instruct them, when they feel their stress levels rise, simply to touch with the index finger of one hand one of the points which I have needled at a recent treatment, at the same time as taking one to three slow abdominal breaths. Points on the hand or wrist are convenient for this, points such as LI4, PC6, HT7, SI3. This brings about a conditioned response of "experiencing the context for relaxation and healing". An important point to make about this is that by these means, we are able to change not just physiology, but behaviour, since when we are relaxed we behave differently in adversity than when we are in a state of tension.

Chapter 3: Concepts and Principles

3.1 Vitality

The Chinese word usually written in Latin script *qi* or *chi*, and pronounced "tsee" or "tshee", is usually translated into European languages as "energy". *Qi* is the central pillar of traditional Chinese acupuncture and its derivatives in the Orient.

Qi is not a single form of "energy": various kinds of it with different physiological functions have been described in the traditional literature. The different forms are said to differ in their density as well as their mobility. For example, blood is a denser form of *qi*, while *Wei/Oe* (defensive energy) is a less dense form. Even very solid tissues, such as bone, may be thought of as highly dense and less mobile kinds of *qi*.

Most often *qi* is associated with the form of energy that "flows" in special channels (often called "meridians") in an organised way along designated courses through the body. This energy is subtle, fluid, and essential for life and health. *Qi* has never been shown to exist using conventional means of detecting physical energy. Therefore I choose to regard this "energy" not as a definite entity or phenomenon. Some practitioners say that they can feel it, and even manipulate it (for example, by inserting needles into the tissues), but I suspect it may be more mythical than mysterious.

My standpoint is that there is not really any occult, "vital energy", no rarefied stuff, that flows through meridians. Nevertheless, I do accept that *qi* is a useful concept, whose beauty and utility lie in its simplicity. I will accept as much so long as we do not regard it as any distinct kind of physical entity, but rather as a composite quality. It is an abstract concept, not an objective entity. Any subjectively appreciable manifestations of what we call *qi* depend on the combined workings of many physiological processes. One kind of subjectively appreciable manifestation of this *qi* is an impression of healthy normalcy which I will call vitality. I do not see *qi* as the source of our vitality, but vitality itself, a nebulous but appreciable quality that is dependent on numerous factors.

How shall I define vitality? It is the organism's potential for producing and maintaining health. Vitality is the only real cure for ill health, any kind of ill health. It is a product of our physiological and psychological processes. Ultimately it depends upon many things, among which: heredity, environment, traumas both physical and psychological, nutrition and hydration, lifestyle habits, happiness and life satisfaction, stress and coping abilities, work and leisure time activities, exercise, rest and relaxation, sleeping patterns, postural habits, personality, attitudes, spiritual attitude and practice.

Obviously vitality cannot be detected directly by machines. As I have defined it in such an abstract way, and as it is the product of such a multitude of factors, some complex in their own right, and some of which are surely unknown, there will never be an instrument for measuring it. However, it can be appreciated qualitatively and subjectively. It is evident in the colour and complexion of the skin, the colour and clarity of the eyes, an impression of psychological poise and attitude, the person's posture and ease of movement, the palpable qualities of the tissues, the sound of the voice, the strength and quality of the pulse. Indeed, there are various qualitative indices of human health which we may appreciate through our senses, and which are indices of vitality.

Conventional Western medicine likes to put states of ill-health in pigeon holes with different labels on them and call them "diseases". Methods of treatment largely involve artificially changing the chemical environment of the diseased tissues (drug therapy) or removing/killing them (surgery, radiotherapy, chemotherapy). If instead, we see the cause of all ill health (no matter what particular label it has been given) in a lack of vitality, a different approach suggests itself which is common to all diseases: to improve vitality. This point of view sees as diseased not the abnormal tissue or the pathophysiological process, but the unhealthy context in which these could develop. Improving vitality means changing the psycho-biological context from one that easily supports disease to one that does not, one that instead promotes health.

I do not here wish to set one system against the other (although there are indeed circumstances in which they are incompatible). Nor would I wish to suggest that acupuncture is a panacea: like any method, it has important limits. Conventional approaches are better for some kinds and circumstances of ill health, a vitalistic approach is better for others. Nevertheless, I do believe that one can only really speak of "cure" in terms of improving the psycho-biological terrain in which disease develops, rather than eliminating each specific, named disease which develops in it.

3.2 Complementary Opposites

I do like the concepts of *Yin* and *Yang*. They are usually regarded as nouns denoting qualities, but are often used as qualitative adjectives. In practice, they may be used as nouns only in the way that the names of the colours may be: "red is a colour", "*Yin* is a quality or principle". They are possibly more usefully employed as descriptors: "*Yin* energy", "solid organs are *Yin*". *Yin* and *Yang* are never absolutes, they always carry only relative value, like such adjectives as light and dark. There are degrees of light. Dull light is *Yin* with respect to bright light but *Yang* with respect to darkness.

Yin and *Yang* qualities relate to each other in dynamic equilibrium. The existence of one depends on the existence of the other. In any entity, animate or otherwise, a shift in the equilibrium in favour of either one of the pair can only proceed so far, stopping short of the extinction of the other. It then swings backwards and forwards with ever decreasing amplitude until a new state of balance is achieved. However, the "balance" is never static, it always involves a state of flux however small or large, of energy, matter or information flow.

Some people may regard the above as so much mumbo-jumbo. But that is true only if you begin to think of *Yin* and *Yang* as things rather than relative qualities. As relative qualities they make sense when applied to physiology. Physiology depends upon the dynamic interplay of opposite influences. This is the very basis of homoeostasis, in which every aspect of our physiology is regulated by a process of neuroendocrine-mediated negative feedback.

An example of a physiological system which can be simply described by *Yin* and *Yang* is the autonomic nervous system (ANS). We could say that the parasympathetic branch (PNS) has a *Yin* function (nurturing) with respect to the more *Yang* (stimulating) SNS. Activation of the former brings about general body maintenance functions (e.g. digestion, anabolism, muscular relaxation), while the latter primes it for action (e.g. cardiocirculatory activation, catabolism, skeletal muscle tensing). Both branches are always active in a dynamic state of equilibrium which shifts according to the diurnal and moment-by-moment needs of the organism.

I believe that so much of what is achievable by acupuncture treatment is achieved through general shifts in the baselines of the major physiological control systems. Such general, longer-term adaptive shifts are known as "allostasis". Acupuncture is above all an adaptogenic treatment, and achieves its effects through general allostatic shifts. As they are such general effects, we do not need to describe their details very exactly or precisely. We do not wish to micromanage physiology. *Yin* and *Yang* are often quite adequate descriptors. They have the advantage of being simple terms which cover many bases, which is one of the general themes of this book.

3.3 Connectivity

Elemental Correspondences

Traditional Chinese medicine proposes that all things can be classified as belonging to one of five basic classes, known as "elements", "movements" or "phases". These are given the names of what were considered the elemental components of the world: Wood, Fire, Earth, Metal and Water. (We will use capitals to indicate that these words have symbolic rather than literal meaning.) The words "movement" or "phase" are perhaps preferable as they imply transformation, one of the universal principles of Chinese philosophy. However, in the following we will use the word "element" as it has gained greater currency in the West.

Thus, the "Water" phase describes the nature of the following things, for example: the kidneys and urinary tracts (and their respective meridians), bone, the ears and hearing, fear, a groaning tone of voice, cold (in general and of the weather), north, winter, black, salty, millet, the pig (and pork), shell-covered animals, black beans. Likewise with all the other phases: they have corresponding bodily organs, meridians, tissues, sense organs, emotions, vocal sounds, types of weather, directions, seasons, colours, grains, animal and vegetable foods, and so on. Each phase also has its own *Yin-Yang* quality: "Water", for instance is "utmost *Yin*".

There are things that strike me as profound and compelling about this system, and other things which strike me as contrived and simplistic. First, the things I like. Above all, some of these correspondences (particularly the ones regarding human biology) are the fruit of long and acute observation and are frequently accurate. To give single examples would arouse accusations of cherry-picking. But examples are certainly not scarce. Anyone with a knowledge of TCM theory as well as human biology, and who has observed the human being for a few years, could quickly think of many.

On the other hand, many of the correspondences seem either arbitrary or too exclusively and rigidly delimited, or both. I imagine the following train of thought playing out among ancient Chinese doctors:

"Our sages tell us that the universe is made of five elements. There are five elements just as there are five senses, five vital bodily organs and five tastes. Indeed we can find some useful relationships between the five components of different classes of things. But if this is a universal principle, everything must follow it. Therefore we must describe all classes of things according to this principle. And it follows that all things will influence each other according to the laws which govern the five elements."

If this is indeed something like their reasoning, it is not good logic. What they ended up with is the dogma of slotting all reality conveniently into an artificial and contrived system of categories. Thus the ear "corresponds" to the kidney and everything in its elemental (or energetic) class - possibly just because of the simple observation that deafness is a corollary of old age (Kidney *qi* is considered a vital quotient that diminishes with age), possibly also because of its "signature": it is shaped a bit like a kidney. I might be understating the point to say that this might not always be the best foundation upon which to build a therapeutic plan. Not that it makes as much difference as purists would like, because so far as systemic effects are concerned, if you put a needle into the spleen meridian instead of the kidney meridian, it makes not a blind bit of difference!

What of the laws which govern the five phases? The two main principles are those of generation and destruction. Wood generates Fire which generates Earth which generates Metal which generates Water (condensation?) which generates Wood again. With a certain amount of imagination one can sort of make an argument for this.

Wood destroys (breaks up? breaks down?) Earth which destroys (absorbs) Water which destroys (puts out) Fire which destroys (melts) Metal which destroys (cuts) Wood. This requires a little more poetic licence, but still, it sort of works. But the problem is that by manipulating the cycle of the five elements and its governing principles in any given case, one can make an argument for almost any diagnosis and almost any treatment plan! And this is, in fact, exactly what different TCM doctors do.

Where do those principles take me in practice? I am told (among other options) that to stimulate the *qi* of the liver meridian I could needle the Water point of that meridian (Water generates Wood); to drain an excess that has invaded that meridian, I could needle its Fire point (as Wood generates Fire, Fire is said to consume Wood). If the excess is not an invasion from outside, but generated within the Wood meridian system, I could instead use the principle of destruction and choose the Metal point (Metal cuts Wood). But my belief is another. My belief is that this is an overly rationalised system: there is no reality in it, beyond the beliefs of its adherents. In a phrase, it is a set of unrealistic folk laws. (By the way, I am not saying and I do not believe that all folk laws are unrealistic, but this one is.)

To be pragmatic, is it useful? Paradoxically yes, in a way, but not in a way that enables me personally. It is useful to many traditional practitioners because it constitutes a framework for a reasoned treatment plan. I believe the reasoning involved to be largely irrelevant to the outcome of the treatment, except for two of its correlates: belief and intent. If the practitioner believes his or her treatment is the right one, he or she is likely to convey a feeling of confidence, as well as a positive intent, to patients, and these are without any doubt important contributory factors to positive outcomes. If the practitioner were reduced to needling acupuncture points randomly there would be no structure on which to hang that belief. An empirical treatment is likely to engender less conviction than an elaborately reasoned one. But for me it is not empowering because I do not believe in it. I have other empowering beliefs about where best to needle and why.

Meridians Are Not Structures and They Have No Biological Functions

I do not believe that there are special channels ("meridians") in the body for the circulation of *qi*. I believe that the organisation of the body's resources is a more complex and less contrived affair than this.

This organisation is controlled by the central nervous system (CNS). It is mediated by information flow, rather than "energy" flow. Information is transmitted by means of nerve impulses, axonal flow, chemical messengers, communication involving components of the immune system, and by mechanical transduction. (There may be other means, some of which as yet unknown, but the word is "information", not "energy".)

Nerves, blood and lymph vessels, and connective tissue planes and networks are the structures by which this transmission is achieved. This is what we know from scientific investigation, which has found no sign of any hitherto scientifically unknown physical structures corresponding either to meridians or to any physiological phenomena that could be uniquely related to such structures[14][15][16][17].

Above I hazarded a guess about the way in which the meridians were afforded specific functions. Similarly, I guess that the whole theory of meridians came into being through a like process of fallacious associations, perhaps such as the following.

People in ancient China noticed that there were certain points on the surface of the body which seemed to be significant either diagnostically or therapeutically. They also noticed that some of the points seemed to be functionally associated in some way or the other, for example in the distribution of pain. One such association they may have observed is the one we know now as myofascial trigger points and their referral areas: an active trigger point can generate pain and activate secondary trigger points in its area of referral. They observed too the distribution of pain or sensory changes occurring in the dermatomal or myotomal territory of spinal nerves, and the phenomenon of visceral referred pain. They observed human anatomy and found organised networks of fascial planes connecting up the body. Then they simply joined the dots, in ways that seemed reasonable to them considering the symptom patterns, the topography, the anatomy, and their world view. I say they seemed reasonable. We must however allow for the human mind's predilection for recognising meaningful patterns even where there is

14 Langevin HM, Yandow JA. Relationship of acupuncture points and meridians to connective tissue planes. *Anat Rec*. 2002;269(6):257-265. doi:10.1002/ar.10185

15 Longhurst JC. Defining meridians: a modern basis of understanding. *J Acupunct Meridian Stud*. 2010;3(2):67-74. doi:10.1016/S2005-2901(10)60014-3

16 Chiang (2015) "...interprets meridian-vessels as neurovascular bundles ... that course beneath connective tissue planes". On Langevin & Yandow's (2002) work, he comments: "Although, Langevin et al.'s research found overlaps between acupoints/merdians and connective tissue planes, the actual relationship is between the peripheral nerves that are underneath". Chiang P. What is the Point of Acupuncture? *Medical Acupuncture*. 2015;27(2):67-80.

17 Li T, Tang BQ, Zhang WB, Zhao M, Hu Q, Ahn A. In Vivo Visualization of the Pericardium Meridian with Fluorescent Dyes. *Evid Based Complement Alternat Med*. 2021;2021:5581227. Published 2021 Mar 29. doi:10.1155/2021/5581227

only randomness (apophenia). The constellations of stars in the night sky is one example of this. Just as the stars in the sky can be connected by imaginary lines to form imaginary constellations, so could the points on the body's surface be connected to form imaginary meridians.

Thus, my contention is that disparate classes of information about body connectivity and a significant dose of fancy combined to produce maps of meridians. The attribution of certain functions to each discrete meridian is in good part a product of people's imagination. The lines, as such, are imaginary: they do not exist either as structures or discrete functional entities. Even though they are supposed to denote functional arrangements, they are merely some kind of map, a rather imperfect one, and not the territory itself. They are like the contour lines showing elevation on a geographical map. If you went to a hill shown on the map and dug for the contour lines, you would not find them, just as you cannot find dedicated *qi* channels in the body.

I do not say this map is without use. Just like contour lines on the cartographer's map, they are indicative of the terrain. One notices on many occasions how they seem to account for some symptom pictures in the way a traditional Chinese physician may have predicted. Why does this person have a cramp-like pain half way down his left calf at the same time as he has pain in his left iliac fossa? There is, currently, a stone passing down his left ureter. I have never seen calf pain described as urinary referred pain in the western medical literature, but to the traditional Chinese physician, it is well established knowledge that the back of the calf is on the urinary bladder meridian. Why has this lady who underwent cholecystectomy 40 years ago had pain affecting her lateral thigh and leg, first on the left, two years later on the right? It is the territory of the gall bladder meridian. The clinical examples are countless.

However, what I say is that the maps of meridians and their points attempt excessive precision, which can easily be interpreted too closely and too literally. It is like confusing a rough rule of thumb with a precise physical law. To practise acupuncture just as effectively and more efficiently, I believe we would do better to refer to more realistic theories about the anatomical and functional arrangements that link the body's surface with its wider workings.

The practice of acupuncture does not necessarily have to refer to the classically described meridian system. In fact I think it can be done without it, more efficiently and at least as effectively. There are two different ways we can manage without meridians. The first is to use acupuncture points or zones for any empirically observable effects they produce. One example of this is the documented stimulation of the Urinary Bladder 67 point to turn a foetus presenting in breach position. The second is to make predictions about which points or zones might produce a desired effect based on what we know about the functional arrangement of the body. Manipulating the flow of *qi* through the meridians, a concept I do not view as realistic, is the traditionally proposed way of doing this. I believe there is a better way.

In another section, we will look at some ways in which the superficial tissues of the body are functionally connected to other areas of the body, and the body as a whole. By "superficial tissues" I mean the skin, the subcutaneous fat, the first few centimetres of muscle, the connective tissue between and among them, ligaments around joints, and the periosteum of accessible bones. These are the tissues into which acupuncture needles are inserted.

3.4 Acupuncture Points

Perhaps naturally enough, the existence or otherwise of acupuncture points has exercised oriental more than occidental minds, so far as scientific attempts at their demonstration are concerned. The Chinese researchers are caught between a culturally determined high regard for tradition, and the modern tyranny of the scientific proof. One might say it is open-mindedness that drives them to question the reality of acupuncture points despite the weight of tradition. Yet I have never read a Chinese study that failed to find suggestive evidence of their existence.

Below I have listed some conclusions from recent studies. Compared to non-acupuncture points, the sites of acupuncture points show:

- 80% correspondence between the sites of acupuncture points and the location of intermuscular or intramuscular connective tissue planes (Langevin & Yandow, 2002[18]).

- Different spectral characteristics under photoluminescence spectroscopy, in particular regarding emissions due to flavin adenine dinucleotide (FAD), phospholipids, and porphyrins (Zhang et al., 2006[19]).

- Elevated concentrations of certain metallic elements (Yan et al., 2009[20]).

- Evidence does not support the claim that acupuncture points are electrically distinguishable from non-acupuncture points (Ahn et al., 2010[21]).

- Higher partial pressure of oxygen (pO2) in tissues close to

18 Langevin HM, Yandow JA. Relationship of acupuncture points and meridians to connective tissue planes. *Anat Rec.* 2002;269(6):257-265. doi:10.1002/ar.10185

19 Zhang Y, Yan X, Liu C, Dang R, Zhang X. Photoluminescence of acupoint "Waiqiu" in human superficial fascia. *Journal of Luminescence. 2006;119-120:* 96–99.

20 Yan X, Zhang X, Liu C, et al. Do acupuncture points exist?. *Phys Med Biol.* 2009;54(9):N143-N150. doi:10.1088/0031-9155/54/9/N01

21 Ahn AC, Colbert AP, Anderson BJ, et al. Electrical properties of acupuncture points and meridians: a systematic review. *Bioelectromagnetics.* 2008;29(4):245-256. doi:10.1002/bem.20403

points (Hong et al., 2012[22]).

- A higher density of micro-vessels a large amount of "involuted microvascular structures" (Zheng et al., 2010[23]; Chenglin and et al., 2014[24]).

In many of the studies purporting to find significant differences between acupuncture points and non-acupuncture points, we find study limitations and weaknesses such as the following cropping up again and again:

- Tissue samples from cadavers.

- Non-human mammalian tissue samples.

- Limited number of points studied.

- Very low numbers of samples.

- Tissue samples chemically preserved.

- No blinding.

- Reporting omissions and deficiencies (e.g. insufficient procedural detail, unclear language).

- I am not competent to express opinions on the validity and reliability of any of the technical devices or methods used, or the appropriateness of the statistical testing, so you may call me a doubting Tom, but I would be quite surprised if there were not deficiencies on those scores as well anywhere in the above studies.

Setting aside these criticisms for a moment, some of the postulated

22 Hong M, Park SS, Ha Y, et al. Heterogeneity of skin surface oxygen level of wrist in relation to acupuncture point. *Evid Based Complement Alternat Med.* 2012;2012:106762. doi:10.1155/2012/106762

23 Zhang D, Yan X, Zhang X, et al. Synchrotron radiation phase-contrast X-ray CT imaging of acupuncture points. *Anal Bioanal Chem.* 2011;401(3):803-808. doi:10.1007/s00216-011-4913-7

24 Chenglin L, Xiaohua W, Hua X, et al. X-ray phase-contrast CT imaging of the acupoints based on synchrotron radiation. *Journal of Electron Spectroscopy and Related Phenomena.* 2014;196:80–84.

differences between acupuncture and non-acupuncture points might not have any functional significance even if they were real. For example, the significance if any of the reported differences in spectral characteristics, pO2 and metal concentrations is obscure.

Other intriguing findings relate to a "novel circulatory system". Deriving from research by Bong-Han Kim in the 1960s, Korean researchers claim to have identified a vascular system with a "specific anatomical and immunohistochemical signature that sets it apart from the arteriovenous and lymphatic systems": the Primovascular System of PVS (Chikly, 2015[25]). Its components, originally thought to correspond to acupuncture meridians and points, are now thought to be so wide-ranging that such close and restrictive mapping is unrealistic. That is, they cannot be said to correspond with traditional acupuncture meridians. The function of the PVS remains a matter of speculation. Research by contemporary Korean researchers led by Kwang-Sup Soh and Byung-Cheon Lee, supporting the existence of the PVS, has not to date been followed up by others.

Is the weight of all the suggestive evidence at all convincing, or is it down to bias and poor experimental design on the part of the researchers? In a literature review Ramey (2000)[26] concluded, "Whatever the clinical efficacy of needling, there is, as yet, no convincing evidence to show that acupuncture points or meridians exist as discrete entities". He also noted, "Many of the studies purporting to have identified acupuncture points or meridians come from China; the role of publication bias in Chinese literature needs

---

25 Chikly B, Roberts P, Quaghebeur J. Primo Vascular System: A Unique Biological System Shifting a Medical Paradigm [published correction appears in J Am Osteopath Assoc. 2016 Apr;116(4):201]. *J Am Osteopath Assoc.* 2016;116(1):12-21. doi:10.7556/jaoa.2016.002

26 Ramey DW. A Review of the Evidence for the Existence of Acupuncture Points and Meridians. *Americam Association of Equine Practitioners Proceedings.* 2000;46:220-224

to be considered in light of the fact that no trial published in China from 1966 through 1995 found a test treatment to be ineffective".

Personally, I am of an open mind regarding the question of whether the traditionally described acupuncture points have in common some distinct anatomical and/or functional characteristics. On a practical level, I tend to the opinion that there are various kinds of points on the body that may become tender and may produce physiological effects when stimulated. I would hazard a guess that the collective of all these points cannot be described by any consistent anatomical or functional features. Also, generally speaking, they are not of fixed size or precisely fixed location, although often their locations are quite consistent.

3.5 Eight Qualities

The eight qualities (or principles) constitute a way of classifying disease processes:

- Interior / Exterior: "exterior" disease is triggered by some external pathogenic influence; "interior" disease starts by some dysregulation intrinsic to the organism. This is an obvious over-simplification. It seems clear to me that most ill-health begins when there is an unfavourable mismatch between the demands placed upon the organism and the capacity of the organism to cope with those demands. That is, all states of ill-health are at the same time "interior" and "exterior". There is however, a legitimate and practical question as to where and how we (physician and patient) can exert the greatest effective leverage.

- Heat / Cold. This is, on the face of it, a fairly simple question about the characteristics of the symptoms and signs. Do they make the patient feel hot or cold? Are they aggravated by heat or cold? Intuitively, are they describable in terms of heat or cold? (E.g. Acid reflux intuitively has a hot quality: "heartburn".) Do they become manifest as palpable heat or cold? Do they become manifest as observable correlates of heat or cold, e.g. reddening, blanching, the blue colour of cyanosis? However, there are complexities. Patients often report that rheumatic pain is aggravated by cold weather, yet some forms, such as rheumatoid, feature episodes of acute inflammation (heat). These contradictions can usually be resolved by distinguishing between an underlying condition and a particular symptom, or between the long-term tendency and short-term manifestations.

- Full (excess) / Empty (deficiency). Fullness results from exterior causes (such as "invasions" of heat, wind, humidity, or cold) or from a primary excess in energy production or accumulation, either globally or locally. Emptiness is caused by a primary deficiency of energy, or by chronic depletion resulting from the body's inadequate efforts to expel an exterior invasion. A similar criticism of this simplification can be made as that levelled against the Interior / Exterior division above.

- *Yin / Yang.* I have spoken about *Yin* and *Yang* in a previous section. Here, it seems to me to be a redundant dichotomy. Or, better, the overarching one. Interior, cold, empty are all *Yin* categories; Exterior, hot, full all *Yang*. Thus *Yin / Yang* comes over and above the other three dichotomies.

Before proceeding, a further note about "exterior" disease is in order here. The traditional notion that disease may be caused by the invasion of the body by pathogenic entities from outside the body conforms well with the modern notion of infection. The ancients, however, did not think in terms of living organisms as the invading agents, but rather in terms of cosmic influences or spirits. These influences, having entered the body, are seen as microcosms of the same influences at work in the outside environment. (And if our defences are weak, they dance to the same tune as those in the outside environment.) They were given the names of their climatic manifestations: Heat, Cold, Damp, Dryness and Wind; and each had an elemental correspondence (Fire, Water, Earth, Metal and Wood respectively). My view is that these notions carry some useful insight at a pathological and diagnostic level, but are not very useful in treatment. That is, I do not believe that a specific selection of points can selectively treat Hot, Cold, Damp, Dry or Wind conditions. The therapeutic effect of needling has nothing to do with its specific effect according to these classifiers, and everything to do with its systemic, adaptogenic effect, and the natural healing drive of the organism.

Interior / exterior, Heat / Cold, and full / excess: Are they useful categories? Yes, I think they are, to an extent, so long as they make us think, rather than lazily or dogmatically popping each case into its pigeon hole. What kinds of questions should we be asking ourselves?

1. How is this person responding to demands, and what are the challenges that have impinged upon his or her health (in the long-term and the short-term contexts)?

2. To what extent do we have effective leverage working with this person's intrinsic life processes?

3. To what extent do we have effective leverage working on demands placed upon this person from outside? ("Demands" means "challenges" of all kinds: biological, meteorological, mechanical, nutritional, social, and so on.)

4. What is likely to be the most effective way to support a regulatory response in this person?

5. To what extent may this person be susceptible to over-

stimulation?

6. Is this person likely to benefit from or be aggravated by stimulating treatments?

7. Is this person likely to benefit from less intense treatments?

3.6 Acupuncture and Sympathetic Activity

The main thesis of this book is that acupuncture works by modifying the stress response. As sympathetic activation is one of the primary phenomena of the stress response, one would then expect to see a moderating effect on this in response to acupuncture treatment.

Various studies (but not all) have shown acupuncture to modulate sympathetic nerve activity in both animals and humans[27][28][29][30]. However, the precise effects shown are inconsistent and evade simplistic interpretations. Preliminary ideas that may be taken from the available literature are that:

- Acupuncture may either increase sympathetic nerve activity or reduce it in the short term.

- Effects may differ depending on the needling technique used, e.g. simple insertion vs. insertion plus manipulation or electrical stimulation; and the intensity of stimulation.

- Effects may differ depending on the depth of needling, e.g.

27 Middlekauff HR, Yu JL, Hui K. Acupuncture effects on reflex responses to mental stress in humans. *Am J Physiol Regul Integr Comp Physiol*. 2001;280(5):R1462-R1468. doi:10.1152/ajpregu.2001.280.5.R1462

28 Middlekauff HR, Hui K, Yu JL, et al. Acupuncture inhibits sympathetic activation during mental stress in advanced heart failure patients. *J Card Fail*. 2002;8(6):399-406. doi:10.1054/jcaf.2002.129656

29 Haker E, Egekvist H, Bjerring P. Effect of sensory stimulation (acupuncture) on sympathetic and parasympathetic activities in healthy subjects. *J Auton Nerv Syst*. 2000;79(1):52-59. doi:10.1016/s0165-1838(99)00090-9

30 Kimura K, Ishida K, Takahashi N, Toge Y, Tajima F. Effects of acupuncture at the ST-36 point on muscle sympathetic nerve activity and blood pressure in normal adults. *Auton Neurosci*. 2017;208:131-136. doi:10.1016/j.autneu.2017.08.009

skin, muscle.

- Effects may be differentiated by region or end-organ e.g. sympathetic activity in nerves innervating muscle tissue, renal sympathetic nerve activity and splanchnic nerve activity may respond differently to acupuncture.

Study designs have generally used single points, single treatments and short follow-up times, so by no means could be said realistically to represent the clinical practice of acupuncture. However, the salient fact is simply that acupuncture does seem to affect sympathetic nerve activity. My thesis (which however I have no proof for) is that it does not matter whether the short-term modulating effect is one of suppression or stimulation: the body's own righting mechanisms will, in the medium term and with sufficient repetition of treatment, respond to these challenges by tending to reset the baseline around which homoeostasis acts to a level closer to normal. Fundamentally, acupuncture has an adaptogenic effect.

3.7 Acupuncture Is Adaptogenic

I use the term "adaptogenic" to refer to something that calls the body to adapt better to the challenges it is facing or may face. The term is borrowed from herbal medicine, where such plants as *Eleutherococcus senticosus* (Siberian ginseng), *Glycyrrhiza glabra* (liquorice) and *Withania somnifera* (ashwaganda) are often considered to have adaptogenic effects.

I have referred previously to "adaptogenic" points and effects. In reality, I believe that acupuncture treatment as a whole can be considered adaptogenic. Within quite a wide range of treatment intensities and individual responsiveness, and in the medium term, acupuncture treatment has neither stimulatory nor inhibitory effects in any absolute sense; it has regulatory, balancing effects. In response to treatment, any affected physiological parameter should be expected, after a blip upwards or downwards, to shift towards normal, whether it was abnormally high or abnormally low to begin with. This is because acupuncture does nothing but induce a self-regulatory response. We, the therapists, are not in command of this as we might sometimes like to believe, we are merely facilitators. The self-regulatory response happens by its own means, in its own time, on its own terms, and by its own path. Variables such as treatment intensity, choice of points, and individual responsiveness may affect the initial response (lasting up to a few days) in one direction or the other, but when this settles, the overall outcome will tend towards the physiological optimum. The major and important exception to this is where a subject of low vitality is given over-stimulatory, over-long, or too frequently repeated treatments, a circumstance which risks overwhelming the organism's efforts to restore balance, and which may result in physiological exhaustion.

3.8 Components of the Proposed Model

3.8.1 Connectivity Reprised

Systemic Effects

Every time we stub our toe, the whole body is affected by it. Every time we insert a needle into the skin and body tissues, the whole body is affected. By neural and humoral pathways the brain receives information about the noxious stimulus and about the physical damage caused to the tissues. The brain's response is both cognitive and physiological. Cognitively, there is mild distress at the small discomfort caused, a focusing of the attention on the location of the needling, and also the positive ("placebo") effect of the hope/expectation of benefit. Physiologically, the neuroendocrine-immune complex is primed for systemic, regional and local responses to stress, in effect, healing responses. These are the reasons why in some cases a needle placed anywhere in the body will produce a beneficial result.

Fascial Networks

Fascial tissues form a complex, integrated, all-encompassing network throughout the body. There is some evidence that mechanical transduction via fascial tissue may be one way in which information is transmitted in the body. Many traditional acupuncture points are situated in alignment with deep fascial planes (epimysium, for instance), or at the junctions of fascial planes. These things suggest that it might be an excellent plan for the acupuncturist to study fascial anatomy rather than, or at least as well as, meridian maps.

Reflex Points and Their Relations

A number of points on the surface of the body have been observed to become tender under certain circumstances, usually involving trauma, over-use, or referred visceral effects. Such points have been described variously as Head's zones, Chapman's "neurolymphatic" reflexes, Jones' tender points, myofascial trigger points and others. All these points tend to be found in fairly constant locations. Each type of point has been described with reference to certain particular properties, real or supposed.

In the 1890s Sir Henry Head described zones of altered skin sensation at relevant spinal cord segments related to diseases of internal organs. Much of the empirical work done on the significance of such reflex areas has been carried out by osteopathic physicians. In the early years of the 20th century Frank Chapman D.O. described tender gangliform contractions located deep to the skin and subcutaneous tissue on the neck, trunk and proximal limbs, related to visceral dysfunction or disease. Later osteopathic physicians believed that Chapman's reflexes were not only of diagnostic significance, but could be manually stimulated to effect targeted reflex physiological. Lawrence Jones' tender points can occur all over the body and each is supposed to be related to a specific kind of dysfunction of an associated joint. That of "acupuncture points" aside, perhaps the description with the greatest scientific support in a therapeutic sense is that of myofascial trigger points. The term was coined by Janet Travell and Seymor Rinzler in the 1950s. Travell and her colleague David Simons later published findings from their extensive studies in a two-volume book, *Myofascial Pain and Dysfunction: The Trigger Point Manual.* Trigger points are tender points, often where a tight band or nodule can be palpated in muscles, which refer pain to other areas, usually distally. They may occur when myofascial tissues have been mechanically over-stressed and occur in predictable locations. Each has its own typical area of referral. They can occur in skeletal muscle or tendon, as well as in ligaments and periosteum.

These various descriptions might be akin to those of the six blind men in the old story, who each attempted to describe an elephant after touching a different part of it[31]. Indeed, as several of the different kinds of points described by different authors have similar locations, and several are also at the locations of classical acupuncture points, it is likely that in many cases they were observing the same phenomena.

---

31 A group of blind men came across an elephant. One touched its trunk and thought an elephant must be like a great worm. Another felt one of its legs and thought an elephant was like a tree. A third touched an ear and thought an elephant was some sort of large-winged bird. And so on. There are many variants of this story, which probably originated in India.

Visceral Reflex Areas

It is well known that visceral disease may present as pain felt near the body's surface. Each internal organ has its characteristic pain referral area. Practitioners of the manipulative and bodywork disciplines know well how a particular kind of muscle hypertonus may originate reflexly from visceral pathology. There is a question in these disciplines as to whether the reflex traffic is largely one-way (visceral to somatic) or equally bidirectional (somatic to visceral as well). Some argue that the viscera may be affected reflexly by somatic dysfunction, and propose manipulation as a means to treat visceral problems on this basis. There is some evidence showing this sort of effect, but not a great deal, and not of the best quality. Conversely, there is a persuasive argument against: it would be evolutionary suicide to allow traumatic injury to the musculoskeletal system to significantly affect the health of the internal organs. On balance, I have come to the view that simple somatovisceral reflexes may explain some of the effects of acupuncture and manipulation, but their importance is probably limited compared to more complex, centrally modulated reflexes and systemic effects mediated by the brain.

Dermatomes, Myotomes and Sclerotomes

The same considerations apply to these. For instance, we know that S1 radiculopathy can cause pain in the back of the calf in a dermatomal/myotomal distribution, but does a needle in the back of the calf help with the back problem on a simple reflex basis? I believe not. I believe that the real situation is both more complex and, happily for acupuncturists, at the same time simpler. It is more complex because the functional neural pathways are complex, not completely mapped, and almost always involve mediation/modulation by the CNS. Trigger point pain referral patterns are one example of this, as they follow no known, simple neural pathways. Another example is when you scratch an itch in one part of the body and, inexplicably, you feel something like a pin prick in another, apparently unrelated part of the body. But it is also simpler, because response to an acupuncture needle piercing the tissues is, fundamentally, a stress and repair response, and as I have noted, there seems to exist quite a basic functional topography when it comes to the stress response.

3.8.2 Empirical Acupuncture Zones and Areas

Later in life Felix Mann, one of the earlier British authors, largely gave up on traditional acupuncture and developed his own system based on "acupuncture areas" and their zones of influence. His book, *Reinventing Acupuncture*[32], is well worth a read. Paradoxically, he was said to be obsessed by Liver 3, which he used an awful lot for a whole range of problems, including "feeling livery". It is indeed a very good point to needle. But as Mann observed, there are certainly areas of the body, not necessarily centred on classical acupuncture points, which seem especially responsive to needling.

3.8.3 Rationale

The theoretical basis of my approach consists of the following propositions:

1. The response to acupuncture is a stress response.

2. The longer-term effects of acupuncture are systemic and mediated primarily by the central nervous system, and secondarily by the endocrine and immune systems.

3. Acupuncture point specificity (meaning the differential effects of different recognised acupuncture points) has been

---

32 Mann F. *Reinventing Acupuncture. A New Concept of an Ancient Medicine.* 2nd edition. Butterworth-Heinemann; 2000.

over-stated.

4. That the body can be divided vertically and horizontally, in a much simpler and more therapeutically functional way than that proposed by the meridian system.

5. The are several major points or "super points" which have greater potency to activate body-wide responses.

Centrally Mediated Systemic Effects

A needle puncturing the skin and underlying muscle is interpreted as a noxious event by the brain. The brain enacts a healing and recuperative response locally, regionally and systemically. This involves an inflammatory response locally and a wider neuroendocrine response affecting many aspects of physiology, e.g. autonomic balance, blood circulation, digestion, metabolism, immunity, tissue repair.

Vertical Connectivity

Vertical connectivity is provided for in part by the segmentally organised "tomes" (dermatomes, myotomes, sclerotomes), in part by the fascial network, in part by myofascial trigger points and their associated referral areas (although the most obvious effects of these are proximal to distal), and possibly in part by as yet unknown systems and phenomena.

Tomes

Myotomes have both sensory and motor innervation, while dermatomes and sclerotomes have only sensory innervation. There are also "vasculotomes" and "viscerotomes". For simplicity, we will just refer to the dermatomes, which are in any case broadly correspondent topographically to the underlying myotomes[33]. In the upper limbs the vertically aligned dermatomes range from spinal segments C5 to T1, and in the lower limbs from L2 to S2.

Now, if one accepts that a sufficient and appropriate stimulus applied in the dermatomal distribution of a spinal nerve may produce reflex effects in the corresponding sympathetic ganglion, these levels would provide for potential effects on the organs and glands of the thorax including the thyroid, the bronchi and the heart; and those of the lower abdomen and pelvis including the last section of the small intestine, the colon and rectum (inferior mesenteric ganglion), the bladder and urinary tracts, and the reproductive apparatus.

However, it seems to be the case that such reflex effects may include levels a little higher and a little lower than those of the afferent stimulus (that is, they may travel a little up and down the cord or sympathetic chain). This widens the range of the potential visceral effects we could achieve from stimulating the sensory nerves in the arms or legs. These effects could be transmitted for example to the parts supplied by the upper cervical ganglion (throat, neck, head and face) and the aorticorenal ganglion (kidneys, adrenals, small intestine).

The organs furthest from these influences are those which receive their sympathetic innervation predominantly from the celiac ganglion (T5 to T9). They are those of the superior abdomen: the liver, gall bladder, pancreas, stomach and spleen.

Let us not forget the parasympathetic, which may potentially be influenced through dermatome S2: descending colon, sigmoid, rectum, urinary bladder, external genitalia.

As I have said, I do not believe these are simple reflex effects, for

---

33 "Hilton's law" observes that the nerve supplying the muscles extending directly across and acting at a given joint also innervate the joint. The law can generally be extended to include the skin over the same muscles and joint.

they are always modulated by stimulatory or inhibitory influences from higher centres. However, as *complex* reflex effects they provide potential pathways for acupuncture intervention.

Fascia

Vertical connectivity is also provided by the fascial planes. The muscles of the limbs run for the most part vertically. Their divisions and subdivisions are formed by connective tissue layers (epimysium, perimysium, endomysium). These fascial layers are part of a continuous connective tissue network that extends throughout the body, comprising myofascia, tendon, ligament and periosteum. By way of example, let us follow one prominent fascial tract for the whole length of the body. This tract arises from the dorsum of the foot via the tibialis anterior tendon, and proceeds through tibialis anterior, the lateral patellar retinaculum, rectus femoris, iliopsoas, the medial arcuate ligament of the diaphragm, the diaphragm itself, the central tendon of the diaphragm, the pericardium, the periostea of the thoracic spine and sternum, the anterior neck myofascia, the periostea of the cranial base and mastoid processes. We should remember also the anatomical proximity and/or continuity of some of these structures with the internal organs, for instance the kidneys which ride on the psoas muscles, and the spleen, stomach, liver and colon which hang from the diaphragm.

Fascia has been shown to posses certain, relatively little known, properties:

- It receives motor innervation and contains contractile fibres.

- It serves as a medium, vector of transport, modulator, and substrate for communication for cells of the immune system.

- It transmits information about mechanical stimuli.

These properties certainly make it look interesting to the acupuncturist.

Myofascial Trigger Points

Generally speaking, when a trigger point on the arms or legs is active, pressure upon it or stimulation with a needle refers pain distally. This is probably different from the vertical connectivity provided by tomes and by fascia. Acupuncturists commonly observe that needle manipulation may cause pain to radiate either proximally or distally.

Combining Tomes, Fascial Planes and Trigger Points

It is my contention that dermatomes, fascial planes and trigger points may go a long way to explaining certain symptom presentations, as well as many of the observable effects of acupuncture. I believe that there are vertically arranged zonal effects, such that the effects of point stimulation are greater if certain general regional correspondences are observed. For example needling the back of the legs is more likely to affect the dorsum of the body and the retroperitoneal organs than the front of the body and the intraperitoneal organs. It can also reach the urinary bladder, urethra, and reproductive organs, possibly via the sacral parasympathetic nerves.

Horizontal Connectivity

Horizontal connectivity is provided for by the same means as vertical connectivity, the difference being that there are more arrangements of a horizontal orientation on the trunk than on the limbs, where the orientation is largely vertical. For example, the dermatomes of the trunk are on the horizontal plane, and there are several horizontally arranged fascial structures (notably the pelvic floor, respiratory diaphragm, the ceiling of the thorax, and the cranial base). Interestingly, trigger point referral areas often display a less vertical arrangement on the trunk than they do on the limbs.

Combining Vertical and Horizontal Connectivity

By combining these two kinds of arrangements one can come up with something like a rough grid reference for where we would like to project the effect of our needling. If this sounds less precise than needling points on meridians, then that is of no matter, for the precision of the latter is illusory, while the relativity of the former affords us flexibility and tolerance of error.

3.9 Acupuncture Response Is a Stress Response

We began this section with a discussion about vitality, and I introduced the idea that vitality is the essence of health. Later I discussed the interplay between the demands or challenges to which the organism is exposed, and its capacity to cope with those challenges effectively. When, for whatever reason, we cannot cope with the demands placed upon us, and we cannot quite quickly restore our normal equilibrium, our vitality is compromised and we begin to decline. We can note here that this notion is very similar to the definition of stress proposed by Lazarus[34]:

Stress arises when individuals perceive that they cannot adequately cope with the demands being made on them or with threats to their well-being.

It is also in line with the three stages of Selye's General Adaptation Syndrome.

Under normal circumstances our vitality is maintained by the

34 Lazarus RS. *Psychological Stress and the Coping Process*. McGraw-Hill; 1966. Lazarus and his co-worker S. Folkman later developed the Transactional Model of Stress. They described stress as "...an imbalance between the demands imposed on the organism, and the capacity of the organism to cope with those demands." (Lazarus RS, Folkman S. *Stress, Appraisal, and Coping*. Springer; 1984.)

interplay of opposite physiological tendencies in numerous biological and psychological processes. In physiology, all of these are regulated by a few great control systems, at or near the top of which stands the ANS with its two complementary branches. I have noted the similarity in concept of this organisation with that of *Yin* and *Yang*. The major primary physiological effect of stress is activation of the SNS, thus producing a relative dominance of the SNS over the PNS.

The connectedness of the organism is emphasised by the fact that the stress response is global (systemic) and coordinated. Healing is a system-wide phenomenon. In acupuncture we have a therapeutic tool that also produces a global, coordinated response. The reason for this is that the insertion of a needle into the body's tissues is treated by the organism as a stressor. The various levels of connectedness which I have highlighted in the preceding paragraphs (fascia, tomes, trigger and reflex phenomena) provide for the provision of a systemic, global response, which also encompasses in an integrated way:

1. A certain degree of regional focusing of the response, mediated by the higher centres.

2. A local response, modulated by the higher centres.

Certain points on the surface of the body become tender under pathogenic or pathological conditions. This tenderness may be regarded as a part of the stress response, whether acute and short-term ("alarm" physiology) or milder and long-lasting ("resistance" physiology). These points are the surface manifestations of the underlying workings of an integrated physiological response. It is not unreasonable to propose that tender points are "just asking" to be stimulated, a stimulation that even in the earliest times may well have been achieved by finger or thumb pressure. Many points that are not currently tender are commonly needled in acupuncture practice either because they are postulated to lie upon energy channels involved in the pathological process, or because owing to their relations they might conceivably produce an effect on that process, or because empirically they have been found to be of benefit in similar cases, or simply because they are listed in traditional point prescriptions. In my view the most solid foundation for needling a point is simply that it is tender, or that its stimulation arouses a regional reaction (e.g. radiating pain in the affected region) as these are the surest signs of alignment with the body's own stress response.

One of the main players in the stress response is the ANS. Acupuncture has been shown to affect SNS activity (and we can assume, by extension, ANS balance) in the short term. I contend that, since acupuncture is an adaptogenic treatment, the medium-term effect accumulated over sufficiently repeated treatments, will be towards a more normal equilibrium, whether the initial effect was stimulatory or inhibitory.

The eight qualities are characteristics of the symptoms, and symptoms, in the early and mid-stages of disease, are attempts by the body to re-establish a vital balance, that is, they are manifestations of a stress response. In relation to this, let me remind the reader of the questions we posed earlier:

1. How is this person responding to demands, and what are the challenges that have impinged on his or her health? In the long-term background and the short-term situation?

2. To what extent do we have effective leverage working with this person's intrinsic life processes?

3. To what extent do we have effective leverage working on demands placed upon this person from outside? "Demands" means "challenges" of all kinds: biological, meteorological, mechanical, nutritional, social, and so on.

4. What is likely to be the most effective way to support a

regulatory response in this person?

5. To what extent may this person be susceptible to over-stimulation?

6. Is this person likely to benefit or be aggravated from stimulating treatments?

7. Is this person likely to benefit from less intense treatments?

By considering the eight qualities we are gleaning clues as to how to support the stress response, whose aim is to re-establish a healthy equilibrium.

In summary, my proposed approach sees disease fundamentally as a stress response, at least in the early and middle stages. Treatment should aim to support this response, acting where we have the greatest leverage with the smallest effective further challenge (needle insertion).

Chapter 4: The Question of Acupuncture Point Specificity

This is the only chapter which I have decided to fully reference, simply because the subject matter is so contentious.

The question of acupuncture specificity is unfortunately highly polarised, with traditionalists affirming the veracity of effective uses as described in the classical texts, and lazy revisionists (not all revisionists are lazy) making facile blanket statements such as: "It doesn't matter where you put the needles". My reflection upon my own experience leads me to believe that:

ACUPUNCTURE POINT SPECIFICITY HAS BEEN
OVERSTATED

Please do not react reflexly or emote viscerally to what has just been stated; it is to be taken it literally as it stands, no more and no less. It is a reasonable statement which merits serious and unbiased consideration.

Traditional and modern textbooks of acupuncture give highly specific indications. For example, McDonald (2020)[35], based on his extensive analysis of ten different authoritative sources, lists the following as accepted indications for LR3.

Main Indications	
Uterine bleeding	Convulsions
Hernia (*shan qi*) [*I believe refers to abdominal and inguinal hernias rather than disk hernias*].	Sore throat
	Cold feet or lower extremities
	Low back pain
Urinary incontinence.	Eye pain
(Continues on next page)	*(Continues on next page)*

---

35 McDonald J. *Acupuncture Point Dynamics*. Volume 1. The Six Foot Meridians. Revised edition. Self-published; 2020.

Main Indications
(Continued from previous page)

Strangury (*Lin syndrome*)
Urinary retention.
Urinary problems in general
Medial ankle pain.
Infantile convulsions
Headache
"Visual dizziness" (*mu xuan*)
[BPPV?]
Pain/fullness in sides
Epilepsy

Pain/retraction of genitals
Post-partum hyperhydrosis
Axillary adenitis
Breast abscess
Mastitis
Vomiting
Haematemesis
Diarrhoea
Abdominal pain or cramps
Depression

Other Indications

Pale face & eyes
Dry throat with thirst
Dryness of upper
oesophageal opening
Swelling of lips
Facial oedema
Hypertension
Thrombocytopenia
"Yin tuberculosis"
Difficult evacuation
Lower abdominal fullness
Dyspepsia
"Thunderous rumblings in the
abdomen"
Hepatitis
Jaundice
Nephritis
Haematuria
"Ejaculation does not stop
during coitus"
Irregular menstruation

Amenorrhoea
"Incessant vaginal discharge
in girls"
"Sudden hernia in children"
"Plague & epidemic diseases
in general"
"Vacuity taxation" (*xu lao*)
*[Chronic deficiency
syndromes?]*
Oedema
Joint pain in extremities
Gout
"Neuralgia of chest, flanks &
loins" *[Intercostal
neuralgia?]*
Spinal pain
Sensation loss of ends of
fingers
Lower leg weakness and pain
[Sciatic radiculopathy?]
Muscle spasm

Indications of acupuncture point Liver 3, adapted from McDonald, 2020.
The text in italics between square brackets is my own.

Now, my contention is not that LR3 fails to treat these symptoms or conditions any better than non-acupuncture points. It is the following:

1. The other major acupuncture points of the lower limb (below the knee) may equally treat a similar list of symptoms or conditions.

2. LR3 may treat the described indications of the other major acupuncture points of the lower limb (below the knee) with similar effectiveness to them.

3. The most important non-local effect of the major acupuncture points is general, not specific, and hence in common to a large degree with other such points.

It is a little more complex than this[36], but this specification will do for the moment to give an idea of my proposition. In a nutshell:

ACUPUNCTURE POINT SPECIFICITY HAS BEEN OVERSTATED

I carried out a literature search designed to dissuade me of this view.

Before I begin with my summary of my findings and interpretations, I have to say this. The majority of acupuncture research comes out of China and there is a major issue with it, which is easily stated: Chinese studies rarely present negative results (personal observation, Tang et al., 1999[37], Vickers et al., 1998[38]). This is a problem because

---

36 For example, as far as specifically located disorders are concerned, LR3 affects (in order of potency) first the ipsilateral foot, then the ipsilateral lower limb, then the lower abdomen, then the upper abdomen, then the rest of the trunk, neck, head and face.

37 Tang JL, Zhan SY, Ernst E. Review of randomised controlled trials of traditional Chinese medicine. *BMJ*. 1999;319(7203):160-161. doi:10.1136/bmj.319.7203.160

38 Vickers A, Goyal N, Harland R, Rees R. Do certain countries produce only positive results? A systematic review of controlled trials. *Control Clin Trials*. 1998;19(2):159-166. doi:10.1016/s0197-2456(97)00150-5

it presents an entirely unrealistic picture and therefore casts legitimate doubt on *any* Chinese study. Such an attitude is no doubt unjust to the genuinely valid studies, but there is no way around this. For this reason Chinese studies do not rank highly in influence in my assessment of the evidence.

Functional Magnetic Resonance Imaging

This century there has been a flurry of functional MRI (fMRI) studies purporting to show specificity in the differential ability of acupuncture points to activate or deactivate different brain regions. 66% of these studies were performed in China (Ke Qui, 2020)[39]. One example: Using fMRI Feng et al. (2011)[40] demonstrated statistically significant differences in functional correlations throughout the entire brain following acupuncture at PC6 compared with PC7 and GB37. The authors speculate broadly about the clinical significance of their findings. With respect to GB37 they write:

> *Compared to GB37, the increased correlations for PC6 were primarily between the prefrontal regions and somatosensory regions, whereas decreased correlations were mainly related with the occipital regions. The occipital regions mainly support vision-related processing. As its name "brightness" implies, GB37 was described as a very effective acupoint influencing multiple vision-related disorders, such as the cataracts, night blindness and optic atrophy.*

39   Qiu K, Yin T, Hong X, et al. Does the Acupoint Specificity Exist? Evidence from Functional Neuroimaging Studies. *Curr Med Imaging.* 2020;16(6):629-638. doi:10.2174/1573405615666190220113111

40   Feng Y, Bai L, Zhang W, et al. Investigation of acupoint specificity by whole brain functional connectivity analysis from fMRI data. *Annu Int Conf IEEE Eng Med Biol Soc.* 2011;2011:2784-2787. doi:10.1109/IEMBS.2011.6090762

Nevertheless, Claunch et al. (2012)[41], in discussing their own study of three very frequently used points - ST36, LI4 and LR3 - point out that there is substantial overlap of brain activation patterns:

The results suggest that although these acupoints are commonly used for anti-pain and modulatory effects, they may mobilize the same intrinsic global networks, with substantial overlap of common brain regions to mediate their actions. Our findings showing preferential response of certain limbic-paralimbic structures suggests acupoints may also exhibit relative specificity.

Huang et al. (2012)[42] carried out a systemic review and meta-analyses of fMRI studies. They conclude:

Brain response to acupuncture stimuli encompasses a broad network of regions consistent with not just somatosensory, but also affective and cognitive processing. While the results were heterogeneous, from a descriptive perspective most studies suggest that acupuncture can modulate the activity within specific brain areas, and the evidence based on meta-analyses confirmed some of these results.

However, I would make three points:

1. Their review reports a quite lot of negative evidence ("results were heterogeneous").

2. There seems to be a lot of overlap in reported brain activation patterns.

3. A few acupuncture points (ST36, LI4, LR3) show much

---

41 Claunch JD, Chan ST, Nixon EE, et al. Commonality and specificity of acupuncture action at three acupoints as evidenced by FMRI. *Am J Chin Med.* 2012;40(4):695-712. doi:10.1142/S0192415X12500528

42 Huang W, Pach D, Napadow V, et al. Characterizing acupuncture stimuli using brain imaging with FMRI--a systematic review and meta-analysis of the literature. *PLoS One.* 2012;7(4):e32960. doi:10.1371/journal.pone.0032960

more extensive brain activation patterns than others.

Ke Qui (2020)[43] agrees that specificity as shown by these studies is relative and may be influenced by numerous study variables:

This review affirmed the existence of acupoint specificity and deemed that the acupoint specificity was relative. Multiple factors such as participants, sample size, acupoint combinations, treatment courses, and types of acupoint could influence the expression of acupoint specificity.

Thus it seems to me that any interpretation based on comparisons of single acupoint studies would be flawed.

There are other problems with all of these studies. Firstly, sample sizes are generally small, meaning the statistical power of the studies is low. According to Wikipedia, this is a criticism commonly applicable to fMRI studies. Other problems are with the statistical procedures used (a dead salmon has been shown to exhibit meaningful brain activity when shown pictures of humans in different emotional states!), the fallacious method of reverse inference when interpreting fMRI results (as individual brain areas often serve multiple purposes), the ability of outcomes to be manipulated by changing software parameters, and the occurrence of software bugs (researchers suggest that owing to a computer bug fMRI results prior to 2015 cannot be relied on) (Wikipedia, n.d.)[44].

In view of the unreliability of the majority of studies owing to their origin (China) or date (prior to 2015), the statistical and procedural weaknesses and flaws, and the speculative nature of their clinical

43 Qiu K, Yin T, Hong X, et al. Does the Acupoint Specificity Exist? Evidence from Functional Neuroimaging Studies. *Curr Med Imaging*. 2020;16(6):629-638. doi:10.2174/1573405615666190220113111

44 Wikipedia Foundation. Functional magnetic resonance imaging. Wikipedia. n.d. Updated May 14, 2022. Accessed May 30, 2022. https://en.wikipedia.org/wiki/Functional_magnetic_resonance_imaging

relevance, frequently based on the fallacious method of reverse inference, I do not feel that much weight can be placed on the fMRI studies so far performed in any rebuttal of the proposal that acupuncture point specificity has been overstated.

One interesting observation, when looking at the images produced by some of these studies, is how certain points - notably ST36, LI4 and LR3 - produce much more widespread activity across the brain than other points. The three mentioned are among the points I call *super points* because of their potency and their wide range of indications.

Laboratory Studies

Tjen-A-Looi et al. (2004)[45] evaluated the influence of electroacupuncture (EA) at various sets of points on the excitatory cardiovascular reflex (measured as changes in mean arterial blood pressure - MAP) and rostral ventrolateral medulla activity evoked by stimulation of chemosensitive receptors in a cat's gallbladder with bradykinin (BK) or direct splanchnic nerve (SN) stimulation. The points stimulated overlie deep or superficial somatic nerves: P5–P6 (overlying the median nerve), LI4 –L7 (overlying branches of the median nerve and the superficial radial nerve), LI6 –LI7 (overlying the superficial radial nerve), LI10–LI11 (overlying the deep radial nerve), S36 –S37 (overlying the deep peroneal nerve), and K1–B67 (overlying terminal branches of the tibial nerves). For clarity I will summarise their findings in bullet points:

- Point-specific differences in magnitude and duration of EA inhibition were observed between P5–P6, LI10–LI11, LI4 – L7 and S36–S37.

---

45 Tjen-A-Looi SC, Li P, Longhurst JC. Medullary substrate and differential cardiovascular responses during stimulation of specific acupoints. *Am J Physiol Regul Integr Comp Physiol.* 2004;287(4):R852-R862. doi:10.1152/ajpregu.00262.2004

- EA at these four sites modulated the sympathoexcitatory pressor responses to gallbladder stimulation by 42, 39, 25, and 32% respectively.

- The degree of modulation of the reflex pressor response was significantly greater with acupoints P5–P6 and LI10–LI11 compared with LI6–LI7, K1–B67, or direct stimulation of the superficial radial nerve.

- The degree of modulation caused by stimulation at P5–P6, LI10–LI11, LI4–L7, and S36–S37 was not significantly different.

- EA at LI6 –LI7 and K1–B67 as well as direct stimulation of the superficial radial nerve did not cause any cardiovascular or rVLM neuronal effects.

- Inhibition by EA at acupoints P5–P6, LI10–LI11, LI4–L7, and S36–S37 lasted for 72+/-10, 60+/-12, 26+/-5, and 24+/-6 minutes, respectively.

- This duration was significantly longer for P5–P6 and LI10–LI11 compared with stimulation at LI4 –L7 or S36 –S37.

These findings to me suggest that:

1. *The degree of specificity shown may be a question of stimulation of deep somatic nerves rather than superficial branches.*
2. *While stimulation of the deep peroneal nerve showed some effect, stimulation over deep somatic nerves on the upper extremities may be more effective for the symptom of reactive hypertension.*
3. *The point combinations which effectively reduce blood pressure all include points which acupuncturists use very frequently because of their clinical effectiveness for a wide range of conditions (P6, LI4, LI11, ST36). I have called these super points.*

A further study on the same subject (Zhou et al., 2005[46]) found that while manual and electrical needle stimulation (at P5-P6) were equally effective in evoking a reflex cardiovascular pressor response, *simple needle insertion without stimulation was ineffective*.

Yong Wang et al. (2012)[47] studied how acupuncture at different points influences local metabolites. They report finding that acupuncture stimulation at ST3, ST21, and ST36 influences mainly plasma micromolecular metabolites closely associated with energy metabolism pathways, whereas stimulation at GB34 affects mainly plasma macromolecular metabolites closely linked to lipid metabolism and transport. Acupoint BL40 had no effect on plasma metabolites. BUT (1) This is a Chinese study and therefore cannot be assumed to be reliable. (2) Sample sizes were small. (3) The authors acknowledge that the high variance of the resulting metabolic profiles is a confounding factor. (4) In order to reach their conclusions the authors performed numerous highly complex mathematical/statistical manipulations on the raw data. Statistical overkill to bolster a weak data set ("damned lies and statistics")? Personally, I cannot have much confidence in this study.

Wang et al. (2015)[48] investigated the capacity of selected acupuncture points to regulate the hypothalamic-pituitary-adrenocortical axis. Specific acupuncture points which modulate the HPA axis were identified. The authors report that:

46 Zhou W, Fu LW, Tjen-A-Looi SC, Li P, Longhurst JC. Afferent mechanisms underlying stimulation modality-related modulation of acupuncture-related cardiovascular responses. *J Appl Physiol (1985)*. 2005;98(3):872-880. doi:10.1152/japplphysiol.01079.2004

47 Wang Y, Wu QF, Chen C, et al. Revealing metabolite biomarkers for acupuncture treatment by linear programming based feature selection. *BMC Syst Biol*. 2012;6 Suppl 1(Suppl 1):S15. doi:10.1186/1752-0509-6-S1-S15

48 Wang SJ, Zhang JJ, Yang HY, Wang F, Li ST. Acupoint specificity on acupuncture regulation of hypothalamic- pituitary-adrenal cortex axis function. *BMC Complement Altern Med*. 2015;15:87. Published 2015 Mar 27. doi:10.1186/s12906-015-0625-4

> *Our results reveal that Shenshu (BL23), Ganshu (BL18), Qimen (LR14), Jingmen (GB25), Riyue (GB24), Zangmen (LR13), Dazui (DU14) and auricular concha region (ACR) are the specificity acupoints; and Gallbladder, Liver and Du Channels were the specificity Channels. The acupoints on Gallbladder Channel and the acupoints innervated by the same spinal cord segments as the adrenal gland demonstrated dramatic effects.*

When one reads their paper however, it turns out this is not quite true. It is not possible to assert from the results that acupuncture points are any more effective than non-acupuncture points, that channels have any relevance, or that points have any specificity beyond the regional or segmentally related.

However, this *is* an interesting study that seems to indicate that:

1. ***Points in the lumbar and low to mid thoracic regions elicited a stress response better than points on the abdomen or extremities.***

2. ***With regard to points on the trunk, the nearer to the spinal segments with sympathetic innervation to the adrenal glands, the greater the response.***

Having said this, I found some of the writing in the results section somewhat convoluted and fatally ungrammatical, so maybe I missed something.

Several other groups have compared the effects of hindlimb versus abdominal stimulation in laboratory animals.

In 1979 a group in Japan studied the neural mechanisms of reflex facilitation and inhibition of gastric motility to stimulation of various skin areas in rats (Kametani et al., 1979[49]). Mechanical nociceptive

---

49 Kametani H, Sato A, Sato Y, Simpson A. Neural mechanisms of reflex facilitation and inhibition of gastric motility to stimulation of various skin areas in rats. *J*

stimulation was delivered to either hind paw or abdominal skin respectively. Hindpaw stimulation produced reflex facilitation while abdominal stimulation produced inhibition of gastric motility. After bilaterally sectioning the splanchnic nerves in vagal intact animals, the reflex facilitation of gastric motility produced by hind paw stimulation persisted, but the reflex inhibition previously produced by abdominal skin stimulation disappeared. Conversely bilateral vagotomy in splanchnic nerve intact animals did not influence the gastric reflex inhibition by abdominal skin stimulation, but either abolished gastric reflex facilitation produced by hind paw stimulation or reversed the reflex facilitation response to slight reflex inhibition. *It was concluded that the gastric reflex facilitation produced by hindpaw stimulation was a vagal effect, while the gastric reflex inhibition produced by abdominal stimulation was effected through sympathetic activation*. After spinal transection at the cervical level, the reflex facilitation of gastric motility previously produced by stimulation of a hind paw was completely abolished, or reversed to slight reflex inhibition, while reflex inhibition of gastric motility produced by stimulation of abdominal skin remained. *It was concluded that the gastric reflex inhibition produced by abdominal stimulation was a spinal reflex*. Simultaneous stimulation of both hind paws and abdominal skin produced partial cancellation of each effect by the other. However, sympathetic reflex inhibition of gastric motility seemed to be much stronger than the vagal reflex facilitatory effect.

Using a genetic technique to ablate a certain type of noradrenergic neurons/adrenal chromaffin cells (NPY+ neurons/cells) Liu et al. (2020)[50] studied the effects of electroactupuncture (EA) on

---

Physiol. 1979;294:407-418. doi:10.1113/jphysiol.1979.sp012937

50 Liu S, Wang ZF, Su YS, et al. Somatotopic Organization and Intensity Dependence in Driving Distinct NPY-Expressing Sympathetic Pathways by Electroacupuncture. Neuron. 2020;108(3):436-450.e7. doi:10.1016/j.neuron.2020.07.015

inflammation induced by endotoxins in mice. They found that low-intensity EA at hindlimb regions drives the vagal-adrenal axis, producing anti-inflammatory effects that depend on NPY+ adrenal chromaffin cells. High-intensity ES at the abdomen activates NPY+ splenic noradrenergic neurons via the spinal-sympathetic axis. This sympathetic activation produces either anti- or pro-inflammatory effects depending on the adrenergic receptor profile, the latter being dependent on disease state. It is important to highlight that these effects were dependent on the intensity of electrical stimulation:

- ***Low intensity at the hindlimb for vagal responses. High intensity did not work.***

- ***High intensity at the abdomen for sympathetic responses. Low intensity did not work.***

Subsequently Lui et al. (2021)[51] found that in mice the presence of PROKR2Cre sensory nerve fibres were crucial for electroacupuncture to activate vagal efferent neurons and to drive catecholamine release from the adrenal glands. These fibres innervate the deep hindlimb fascia (for example, the periosteum) but not abdominal fascia (for example, the peritoneum). The authors comment:

> *We argue that acupoint specificity, which has been long debated in the acupuncture field is an operational definition that depends on the stimulation intensities, the depth at which the needle is placed and the outcomes measured. For example, for low-intensity ES [electroacupuncture stimulation], deep but not superficial stimulation of the ST36 site is crucial for driving the vagal–adrenal axis, which probably reflects the requirement of electric needle tips close*

---

51 Liu S, Wang Z, Su Y, et al. A neuroanatomical basis for electroacupuncture to drive the vagal-adrenal axis [published correction appears in Nature. 2022 Jan;601(7893):E9]. *Nature.* 2021;598(7882):641-645. doi:10.1038/s41586-021-04001-4

> *to the major nerve bundles containing PROKR2ADV fibres that innervate deep limb fascia ... By contrast, spinal sympathetic reflexes, which are independent of PROKR2ADV neurons, can be evoked by high-intensity ES at both ST25 and ST36 acupoints.*

I am happy with their assessment. Point specificity as such has been overstated. **Specific effects are contingent on the fulfilment of conditions beyond point selection.** Nevertheless, there seems to be a clear difference in the effects of hindlimb versus abdominal stimulation. I envisage that it will be found that this is generalisable to all limbs versus trunk.

Continuing with the theme of rodent hindlimb stimulation, Quiroz-González et al. (2014)[52] investigated the distribution and amplitude of cord dorsum potentials (CPDs) produced by EA at (a) acupuncture points on the GB and BL meridians, (b) non-acupoint sites on the same meridians, and (c) non-meridian sites. They found that:

1. Stimulation produced CPDs over several segments, peaking at one segment.

2. Non-acupoint sites on the same meridians produced similar CPD distributions and amplitudes as the acupoints.

3. Non-meridian sites produced CPDs with similar distributions but of smaller amplitude than acupoints.

These results are consistent with notions of potency of effect and <u>relative</u> specificity. There would seem to be longitudinally organised areas ("meridians") of greater potency than surrounding areas. I expect further research will find them to be less well-defined than the meridian model would suggest.

---

52 Quiroz-González S, Segura-Alegría B, Guadarrama-Olmos JC, Jiménez-Estrada I. Cord dorsum potentials evoked by electroacupuncture applied to the hind limbs of rats. J Acupunct Meridian Stud. 2014;7(1):25-32. doi:10.1016/j.jams.2013.06.013

An interesting Korean study on cocaine addiction in rats was carried out by Jin et al. (2018)[53]. Cocaine suppresses the release of the neurotransmitter gamma-Aminobutyric acid (GABA) in the ventral tegmental area (VTA) of the midbrain. The authors report that acupuncture at HT7 significantly reduced cocaine suppression of GABA activity in the VTA. HT7 acupuncture also attenuated cocaine-primed reinstatement of cocaine-seeking behaviour. Cocaine increases dopamine release in the nucleus accumbens (NAc) and repeated intake increases this effect. This is related to increased cocaine-seeking behaviour, a phenomenon known as behavioural sensitisation. HT7 acupuncture attenuated cocaine-induced behavioural sensitisation by inhibiting dopamine release in the NAc. Moreover, acupuncture at HT7 reduced acute cocaine-induced locomotor activity and neuronal activation in the NAc *in a depth-dependent fashion*.

Critically, the researchers compared the effects of HT7 acupuncture with LI5, PC5 and a non-acupuncture control point on the rat's tail. *The reversal of cocaine-induced inhibition of GABA release in the VTA was active when needling HT7, but not when needling LI5. Also, the reinstatement of cocaine-seeking behaviour was reduced by HT7 but not LI5.* Further, *acupuncture at HT7, but not at PC6, reversed behavioural sensitisation by decreasing the excessive dopamine levels caused by cocaine intake.*

The limitations of this study are:

1. The authors do not discuss the limitations of their study.

2. The authors report the way in which HT7 is inserted, to what depths and with what kind of stimulation, but they do not report the same information for their alternative treatment

---

53 Jin W, Kim MS, Jang EY, et al. Acupuncture reduces relapse to cocaine-seeking behavior via activation of GABA neurons in the ventral tegmental area. *Addict Biol*. 2018;23(1):165-181. doi:10.1111/adb.12499

points or the control point. One is left to assume (hope?) they were treated in the same general way.

3. With regard to the reversal of cocaine-induced inhibition of GABA release in the VTA, the authors report the results of HT7 compared with LI5, but not with PC6.

4. With regard to the reinstatement of cocaine-seeking behaviour, similarly the authors report the results of HT7 compared with LI5, but not with PC6.

5. With regard to the reversal of behavioural sensitisation, the authors report the results of HT7 compared with PC6, but not with LI5.

One is left with the doubt that reporting may have been selective in order to strengthen the proposition that acupuncture's effects on cocaine addiction are highly specific to HT7. Whereas in fact for two of the measured outcomes the effects of PC6 may not be significantly different, and for the third those of LI5 may be of equivalent magnitude. We do not know, because the results were not fully reported!

Nevertheless, HT7 does seem to have partial specificity in this regard, and its effects are needle-depth dependent. This leads the authors to postulate that:

... the ulnar nerve originating in the skin and muscle is involved in the peripheral sensory mechanisms of HT7 acupuncture. Given afferent signals during acupuncture, the present results suggest the possibility that HT7 acupuncture at deep tissue may recruit more A-fibers within the ulnar nerve than that at superficial tissue. This may result in greater responses.

This is one of several studies to suggest that **the distant and systemic effects of acupuncture are achieved by** *recruitment of*

deep somatic nerve fibres.

It should be noted that results from many of the above studies come from mutilated anaesthetised laboratory animals not closely related phylogenetically to *homo sapiens*, and so not necessarily generalisable to live members of our species in a normal clinical setting.

Clinical Trials

In a review paper Jing-jing Xing et al. (2013)[54] report on a study by Li et al. (2008)[55] thus:

> *A ... multicenter study of 480 patients with migraine was participated, investigating long-term analgesic effect between acupoints and nonacupoints and exploring the differences between different acupoints (Li et al., 2008). The patients were randomized into treatment group 1 (Shaoyang-specific acupuncture), treatment group 2 (Shaoyang-nonspecific acupuncture), treatment group 3 (Yangming-specific acupuncture), and the control group (nonacupoint group). After 4 weeks' treatments, the primary outcome, which was the number of days when the subjects experienced a migraine during weeks 4–8 and 13–16, was assessed. Fewer days with migraine were witnessed in three acupuncture groups compared with nonacupoint group during weeks 4–8, and with no difference between treatment groups (P > 0.05) and significant fewer days during weeks 13–16 (Shaoyang-specific acupuncture vs. control (P < 0.01); Shaoyang-nonspecific acupuncture vs. control (P <*

54 Xing JJ, Zeng BY, Li J, Zhuang Y, Liang FR. Acupuncture point specificity. *Int Rev Neurobiol*. 2013;111:49-65. doi:10.1016/B978-0-12-411545-3.00003-1

55 Li Y, Liang F, Yu S, et al. Randomized controlled trial to treat migraine with acupuncture: design and protocol. *Trials*. 2008;9:57. Published 2008 Oct 20. doi:10.1186/1745-6215-9-57

0.01); Yangming-specific acupuncture vs. control (P < 0.05)).

The review authors comment:

This study shows that acupoints are more effective than nonacupoints and acupoints from shaoyang meridian are more effective than Yangming meridian in long-term analgesia for migraine which further presents differences between acupoints and nonacupoints, as well as among acupoints.

Except it doesn't. The reported results indicate that while we we can be 95% certain that Yang Ming acupuncture is effective, we can be 99% certain that Shao Yang acupuncture is. *Significance level and confidence level are measures not of degree of effect but of the probability that the finding of effectiveness is true.*

Secondly, the Li et al. (2008) paper is not a completed study but a study proposal. It does not report any such findings. In fact, there is no 2008 paper on this subject. I eventually found the study referred to (Li et al., 2012[56]). The actual study authors do not say:

"acupoints from shaoyang meridian are more effective than Yangming meridian"

They say:

Compared with patients in the control group, patients in the acupuncture groups reported fewer days with a migraine during weeks 5–8, however the differences between treatments were not significant (p > 0.05). There was a significant reduction in the number of days with a migraine during weeks 13–16 in all acupuncture groups compared with control (Shaoyang-specific acupuncture v. control:

---

56 Li Y, Zheng H, Witt CM, et al. Acupuncture for migraine prophylaxis: a randomized controlled trial. *CMAJ*. 2012;184(4):401-410. doi:10.1503/cmaj.110551

difference –1.06 [95% confidence interval (CI) –1.77 to – 0.5], p = 0.003; Shaoyang-nonspecific acupuncture v. control: difference –1.22 [95% CI –1.92 to –0.52], p < 0.001; Yangming-specific acupuncture v. control: difference – 0.91 [95% CI –1.61 to –0.21], p = 0.011). We found that there was a significant, but not clinically relevant, benefit for almost all secondary outcomes in the three acupuncture groups compared with the control group. We found no relevant differences between the three acupuncture groups.

Note also that the p values reported by the original authors are different from those reported by the review authors. Yet from their description this is surely the study referred to by Jing-jing Xing et al.

I find that skewed reporting/interpretations or clear misreporting crop up with fair frequency in acupuncture papers. Anyway, if the reader has become confused, the outcome was that there was no difference in effectiveness in the treatment of acute migraine between acupuncture on Shaoyang or Yangming points or whether or not the points were considered specific for migraine.

One (Chinese) study that does seem to have shown relative specificity was published by Yang et al. (2012)[57]. It is similar to the previous study in that it compares acupuncture treatment of the Shao Yang channels with that of the Yang Ming channels for migraine. Different groups of patients with migraine were given acupuncture treatment either at TE5, GB34, GB20 (labelled the "Traditional Acupuncture Group" or TAG), LI6, ST36, ST8 (the "Control Acupuncture Group", CAG) or no treatment ("Migraine Group", MG). A single 30 minute electroacupuncture treatment was given to the TAG and CAG during a migraine attack and positron emission tomography with computed tomography (PET-CT) was used to show

---

57　Yang J, Zeng F, Feng Y, et al. A PET-CT study on the specificity of acupoints through acupuncture treatment in migraine patients. *BMC Complement Altern Med.* 2012;12:123. Published 2012 Aug 15. doi:10.1186/1472-6882-12-123

areas of brain activation before and after treatment. Subjects also rated their pain on a visual analogue scale (VAS) before and after treatment. Both TAG and CAG reported diminished pain after treatment and the difference was significant, whereas there was not a significant difference in the MG group. The reduction was greater in the TAG than the CAG. Both the TAG and CAG showed differences in brain glucose metabolism after treatment compared to the MG. The differences affected more areas in the TAG compared to the CAG. This seems to be a well designed study which however suffers from the common weakness of small sample size and therefore low statistical power, and the limitation that it measures only the immediate effects of a single treatment. It remains to be seen whether such effects can be confirmed in larger studies and maintained over the medium term. The Li (2012) paper above would suggest perhaps not.

In another study Yu et al. (2010)[58] compared the immediate effect of acupuncture at SP6 on uterine arterial blood flow in primary dysmenorrhoea (PD) with that of GB39 in 66 patients. Their results suggest that needling at SP6 can immediately improve uterine arterial blood flow of patients with primary dysmenorrhoea, while GB39 does not have these effects. Again I would argue that the effect observed may have more to do with the power of SP6 to produce generalised physiological responses rather than symptom, organ or pathology-specific effects. It is also possible that in addition we are dealing with regional-specific effects (rather than symptom, organ or pathology-specific ones) e.g. medial rather than lateral leg. The authors comment:

> *These different effects of SP6 and GB39 preliminarily show that the specificity of SP6 might be more related to*

---

58 Yu YP, Ma LX, Ma YX, et al. Immediate effect of acupuncture at Sanyinjiao (SP6) and Xuanzhong (GB39) on uterine arterial blood flow in primary dysmenorrhea. *J Altern Complement Med.* 2010;16(10):1073-1078. doi:10.1089/acm.2009.0326

traditional acupuncture meridians rather than other factors such as its innervations and anatomical location.

Might. Also might not. But given that some degree of specificity appears to exist, I would still question the above statement. Firstly the skin and myofascia at SP6 and GB39 are innervated by different segmental levels, with GB39 (L5/S1) receiving innervation from lower segments than SP6 (L4). It is known that sensory information may produce reflex effects from several segments above or below the input segment. Efferent sympathetic flow to the uterus is from T1-L1, which is nearer to L4 than it is to L5/S1. However, I would argue that local reflexes are probably far less important to acupuncture effect than centrally mediated/modulated ones. As to anatomical location, I am of the view that points on the medial leg may have greater effects on the pelvic organs than points on the lateral leg: there is a degree of zonal specificity. So my research question would be: In this context is SP6 any better than KI7 or LR8, for example?

Ma et al. (2010)[59] studied the immediate effect on uterine blood flow and pain of SP6 as compared to GB39 and an adjacent non-meridian point in 50 PD patients. The authors conclude that:

EA at SP6 can immediately relieve menstrual pain and minimize the influence of pain on daily life compared with GB39 and an adjacent non-meridian point. The data preliminarily show the specificity of SP6 for the immediate pain relief of primary dysmenorrhea.

Even though only one of the three primary outcomes was significantly different (the others were measures of uterine blood

---

59 Ma YX, Ma LX, Liu XL, et al. A comparative study on the immediate effects of electroacupuncture at Sanyinjiao (SP6), Xuanzhong (GB39) and a non-meridian point, on menstrual pain and uterine arterial blood flow, in primary dysmenorrhea patients. *Pain Med.* 2010;11(10):1564-1575. doi:10.1111/j.1526-4637.2010.00949.x

flow, which contrary to the Yu et al. 2010 study showed no difference between the points treated), the sample size was small, and the study comes out of China, this is interesting, but again may be explained by the general rather than the specific power of SP6.

It is a pity then that in a larger RCT with 200 PD patients Liu et al. (2011)[60] found that there was no significant difference in pain relief of dysmenorrhea between SP6- and GB39-treated groups. They report:

> *Acupuncture was better than no acupuncture for relieving the pain of dysmenorrhea following a single point of acupuncture, but no differences were detected between acupoint acupuncture and unrelated acupoint acupuncture, acupoint acupuncture and nonacupoint acupuncture.*

I need to point out that (despite the paper's title) whereas the previously described studies measured only immediate effects, this one aimed to measure effect both during treatment and over two menstrual cycles after treatment.

In a study of chronic stable angina Zhao et al. (2019)[61] compared the effect of acupuncture on the "disease-affected meridian" (DAM) with acupuncture on a non-affected meridian (NAM), sham acupuncture (SA), and waiting list (WL = no treatment). PC6 and HT5 were treated in the DAM group and LU9 and LU6 in the NAM group. The DAM and NAM groups received both electrical and robust manual needle stimulation to achieve the *deqi* sensation. The SA group received electrical stimulation but no manual needle

60 Liu CZ, Xie JP, Wang LP, et al. Immediate analgesia effect of single point acupuncture in primary dysmenorrhea: a randomized controlled trial [published correction appears in Pain Med. 2011 Apr;12(4):685]. *Pain Med.* 2011;12(2):300-307. doi:10.1111/j.1526-4637.2010.01017.x

61 Zhao L, Li D, Zheng H, et al. Acupuncture as Adjunctive Therapy for Chronic Stable Angina: A Randomized Clinical Trial. *JAMA Intern Med.* 2019;179(10):1388-1397. doi:10.1001/jamainternmed.2019.2407

manipulation. The authors report that compared with acupuncture on the NAM, SA, or no acupuncture, acupuncture on the DAM as adjunctive treatment to antianginal therapy showed superior benefits in alleviating angina. Improvements over the WL were of similar magnitude between the the NAM and SA groups.

To me this study suggests that *acupuncture with deqi on the anteromedial side of the forearm is more beneficial for heart symptoms than acupuncture on the radial side or acupuncture without deqi. This is consistent with a model that defines acupuncture target-specificity in terms of (a) active regions or zones; (b) point potency. It also highlights the importance of achieving a sufficient intensity of needle stimulation*.

It is worth noting, although real vs. sham acupuncture is not my primary concern, that:

> *Several large-scale randomized controlled trials (RCTs) in chronic pain patients failed to display specificity in acupuncture treatment. Studies include chronic low back pain, fibromyalgia, migraine, and tension-type headache, and the authors found that there was no significant difference of analgesia between verum and sham acupuncture-treated groups* (Jing-jing Xing et al., 2013[62]).

The studies referred to are from 2005 and 2006. It is worth emphasising the words "large-scale" (which increases their power), and I will add that these were all European studies rather than Chinese (which in my view increases their reliability as already noted).

---

62 Xing JJ, Zeng BY, Li J, Zhuang Y, Liang FR. Acupuncture point specificity. *Int Rev Neurobiol.* 2013;111:49-65. doi:10.1016/B978-0-12-411545-3.00003-1

Other Work

In a fascinating study Lee and Chae (2020)[63] used a statistical technique called network analysis to identify major traditional acupuncture points used for pain control in a number of common kinds of painful condition. The most commonly used points were found to be ST36, SP6, LR3, GB34, LI4; the most common point combinations used were SP6–LR3, ST36–GB34, SP6–ST36, LR3–LI4, LR3–ST36. I have included this study here because it confirms the validity of my notion of major (or "super") points, in that the points found to be most used for pain are those that are also most cited for a wide variety of conditions.

This is again born out by Hwang et al. (2020)[64] who analysed acupuncture point selection in clinical trials. They found that the acupuncture points selected for the widest variety of conditions were SP36, ST36, LR3, LI4, GV20.

Similarly Yoo et al. (2022)[65], again using network analysis found that the most common points used in both current practice (based on the Cochrane Database of Systematic Reviews) and ancient practice (based on the ancient medical text Donguibogam) were ST36, SP6, LR3, LI4, and GV20. Acupoints CV3, CV4, CV6, CV8, and CV12 were more widely used in ancient acupuncture, while in current acupuncture, HT7, PC6, KI3, GB34, and EX-HN3 (Yintang) were more prevalent.

---

63 Lee IS, Chae Y. Identification of major traditional acupuncture points for pain control using network analysis. *Acupunct Med.* 2021;39(5):553-554. doi:10.1177/0964528420971309
64 Hwang YC, Lee IS, Ryu Y, Lee YS, Chae Y. Identification of Acupoint Indication from Reverse Inference: Data Mining of Randomized Controlled Clinical Trials. *J Clin Med.* 2020;9(9):3027. Published 2020 Sep 20. doi:10.3390/jcm9093027
65 Yoo Y, Ryu Y, Lee IS, Chae Y. Diachronic analysis of major acupoints used in ancient and current acupuncture treatments: Changes in main acupoints over time. *Integr Med Res.* 2022;11(3):100865. doi:10.1016/j.imr.2022.100865

Choi et al. (2012)[66] carried out a review of studies on acupuncture specificity. I mention it here because it is a good review and because one of the authors was the late John C. Longhurst, a highly regarded scholar. However, it does not add significant information beyond what has already been covered in this chapter. They comment as follows:

> *...many acupuncture studies using this principle* [of acupuncture specificity] *to select control points have found that sham acupoints have similar effects to those of verum acupoints. Furthermore, the results of pain-related studies based on visual analogue scales have not supported the concept of point specificity. In contrast, hemodynamic, functional magnetic resonance imaging and neurophysiological studies evaluating the responses to stimulation of multiple points on the body surface have shown that point-specific actions are present.*

I have already commented on the most significant of those haemodynamic, fMRI and neurophysiological studies in the preceding paragraphs.

In response to my expressed view that acupuncture point specificity had been overstated, an illustrious colleague urged me above all to look at the studies of Poney Chiang, adjunct professor and founding director of the Integrative Acupuncture Certificate Program for the Faculty of Health at York University in Toronto, Canada. Chiang and co-workers carried out a series of studies using dissection and electro-stimulation to map peripheral acupuncture points against

---

66 Choi EM, Jiang F, Longhurst JC. Point specificity in acupuncture. *Chin Med.* 2012;7:4. Published 2012 Feb 28. doi:10.1186/1749-8546-7-4

specific neuroanatomical structures (peripheral somatic nerves)[67][68][69][70][71]. Let us let pass the fact that in order to demonstrate specificity, the authors had to redefine the positions of many acupuncture points because they "missed the ... neuroanatomical target" described by standard texts, or "lacked anatomical precision" in that regard[67]. Ignoring these manipulations, their studies are well and good, but they tell us nothing concrete about the proximal effects of acupuncture point stimulation, only distal effects on muscle action (effects which I class as local). It is worth repeating that my interest is in non-local effects.

However, in "What is the Point of Acupuncture"[67], Chiang makes some interesting assertions:

> *Although the data from the current study partially supports the association between peripheral nerves and meridians, it does not exclude a vessel-based perspective of meridians.*

And:

> *The current author interprets meridian-vessels as neurovascular bundles (Jing Mai) that course beneath connective tissue planes.*

67 Chiang P. What is the Point of Acupuncture? *Med Acupunct.* 2015;27(2):67-80. https://doi.org/10.1089/acu.2015.1093

68 Lee M, Chiang P. A Revised Neuromyofascial Understanding for the Neck, Head and Facial Channel Sinews based on the Ling Shu. *JCM.* 2017;114:34-50.

69 Ortiz D, Chiang P. Neuroanatomical Significance of Acupuncture Points TE1–TE10 Based on the Systematic Classic. *Med Acupunct.* 2017;29(2):66-76. https://doi.org/10.1089/acu.2017.1221

70 Lee M, Longenecker R, Lo S, Chiang P. Distinct Neuroanatomical Structures of Acupoints Kidney 1 to Kidney 8: A Cadaveric Study. *Med Acupunct.* 2019;31(1):19-28. doi:10.1089/acu.2018.1325

71 Meltz L, Ortiz D, Chiang P. The Anatomical Relationship Between Acupoints of the Face and the Trigeminal Nerve. *Med Acupunct.* 2020;32(4):181-193. doi:10.1089/acu.2020.1413

If he is right, then the proximal effects of peripheral acupuncture should be explained in terms of (a) innervation (segmental innervation so far as the neck, trunk and pelvis are concerned); (b) the latter's potential effects on circulatory dynamics; (c) central modulation of (a); (d) centrally generated systemic effects. But these would not be sufficient to provide for the array of specific proximal or distant effects attributed to some acupuncture points, such as LR3 (see the table at the beginning of the chapter).

Conclusions

I find studies on acupuncture point specificity to be plagued by mis-reporting, selective reporting, slanted interpretation, and dubious reliability and/or validity.

The majority of fMRI studies which show acupoint specificity are unreliable (because of their origin, date of publication, statistical and procedural weaknesses and flaws), frequently based on the fallacious method of reverse inference, and speculative as to their clinical relevance.

As regards laboratory, clinical and other studies, across study types, there are points which are utilised time and time again: points such as ST36, LI4, LR3, SP6, GB34. The effects noted may be explained by their special power to produce a generalised response. This is a simpler explanation than that of differential specificity, and therefore the one that should more readily be accepted according to the principle of parsimony (Occam's razor).

The desired proximal effects appear to be more readily produced:

1. By needle insertion over deep somatic nerves rather than superficial branches.

2. By needle insertion into fascia.

3. With needle stimulation (electrical or manual) rather than without.

4. According to some evidence, by stimulation of a specific side of the limb e.g. medial vs. lateral hindlimb, ulnar vs radial side of the arm.

Differential effects are produced by limb versus abdominal stimulation. In rats, gastric facilitation from hindpaw stimulation was a vagal effect, while gastric inhibition from abdominal stimulation is effected through sympathetic activation. The effect is also dependent on the intensity of stimulation, for hindpaw vagal responses, low intensity; for abdominal sympathetic responses, high intensity.

There is some evidence to suggest that especially with regard to acupuncture on the trunk, that greater effects are achieved by the stimulation of points nearer the segmental level involved.

Specific effects are contingent on the fulfilment of conditions beyond point selection.

The results of these studies are consistent with a model that defines acupuncture target-specificity (a) in regional and systemic terms; (b) with reference to neuroanatomy; (b) in terms of point potency. They also highlight the importance of achieving a sufficient intensity of needle stimulation.

84

Chapter 5: Treatment

5.1 Some Pearls of Chinese Medicine

Having read up to this point, the reader might have gained the impression that I have little time for tradition, but this is not true. I have great respect for tradition, but little time for dogma. The history of acupuncture is the story of many, many practitioners down through the ages, the best of whom each took ownership of their discipline by dissecting it, putting it back together again, and using it in their own way. The forthright or influential among them then challenged, fed back into, and modified the prevailing orthodoxy, sometimes with minor tweaks, other times with major new propositions, changes in emphases, or wholesale rejections of the parts they did not find to be true. Different schools formed with different orthodox teachings, but none of them should ever be seen as being set in stone. So in this, what I am doing here is no different from what many, many other practitioners have done before.

Let me add that there are aspects of traditional teachings which I not only accept but hold in awe, and others which I see no reason to reject. Above all I admire:

- The fundamentally and uncompromisingly holistic nature of traditional Chinese medical theory. That its actual practice may often have been pragmatic and empirical does not diminish the holistic philosophy on which it is founded.

- The building of empirical findings into a systematic body wedded to holistic philosophical principles, to produce the simple intricacy found in many schools of traditional oriental medicine, is a masterpiece of the human intellect.

- That notwithstanding my misgivings about traditional Chinese medical theory and practice, the use of acupuncture together with moxibustion and herbal treatment has delivered an effective healthcare system to millions of people for thousands of years.

- The application of truly insightful powers of observation that led to the development of detailed descriptions of a wide range of recognised syndromes and corresponding diagnostic signs.

- Pulse diagnosis. Some readers may raise their eyebrows at this. I have been sceptical of so much, why not this most subjective and scientifically implausible of methods? My experience is that it can be remarkably helpful, but it is subjective and unreliable across practitioners. It is perhaps not for everyone. I have my own theory about it, which I have already touched upon.

5.2 General Philosophy

I believe the primary role of acupuncture is in the treatment of conditions that lie more on the "functional" than the "organic" side of pathology. Certainly, it is in this field that it comes into its own and it is here that conventional medicine consistently demonstrates its limitations. Important then is the need for us to understand pathology as a dynamic and evolving process, so that we may recognise it at its earliest stages and apply corrective measures while they may best be influential: while the adaptive, recuperative mechanisms are still intact or retrievable.

Perceived adversity produces neuroendocrine responses in order to bring about physiological adaptations to that adversity. This is the basis of the body's stress response. These neuroendocrine responses involve the autonomic nervous system and the hypothalamus-pituitary-adrenal (HPA) axis. A cornerstone of the physiological stress response is the sympathetic nervous system. Sympathetic activity and adrenergic endocrine activity stimulate and enhance each other.

I am of the opinion that excessive and/or inappropriate sympathetic-adrenergic activation is one of the greatest causes of ill-health in modern societies. Autonomic balance is determined principally by this. Parasympathetic activity will largely look after itself, if not inhibited or dysregulated by maladaptive sympathetic activation. This is a fundamental basis of much pathology.

A maladaptive or prolonged stress response will cause dysfunction in all physiological systems, but it will do so most where it impacts upon our weakest links, whether that prior weakness be determined by heredity or environmental factors.

In this context, what is the most rational therapeutic response? With regard to the weakest link (whether it be the stomach, the colon, the lungs, the liver, etc.) it must be rested and nourished, not stimulated. It must be given an environment that promotes vitality rather than degradation. That means it needs a good blood and nerve supply and good blood and lymphatic drainage. The blood must supply what is needed, so it must receive from the gut the right nutrients, which must have been processed well by the liver. The blood must not be full of wastes and toxins, so the liver and kidneys must be working effectively. Oxygen and carbon dioxide must be present in the blood in the right mix, so the tissues are well oxygenated and bathed in fluids at optimal pH. Thus the lungs must be healthy and breathing patterns normal. It is easy to see how this quickly becomes a global problem, not just a problem with a symptomatic organ.

The answer is simply stated: we must work to reduce sympathetic-adrenergic activation by any means, combining acupuncture as needed with, for instance, manual treatment, herbs, cognitive-behavioural therapy, encourage nurturing habits and beneficial behaviours in diet, hydration, sleep and rest, activity, breathing and postural patterns, relationships and socialisation.

This kind of general approach, using acupuncture as a tool rather than the be-all-and-end-all, removes symptomatic treatment to a secondary level, except in acute cases, if indeed it is necessary at all. It is well to remember that improving general health is the only real chance of cure for any illness.

5.3 Overarching Principles

In this context of a stress-based model, I wish to state here four general, functional principles of treatment.

- Firstly, we can neither give nor take away energy or resources with a needle. What we can do is to stimulate the body to use its vital energy to create a better context for healing, and, to a certain extent, direct its healing attention to areas of need. But we cannot do this in the very specific way in which many practitioners like to believe they operate.

- Secondly, the most important mechanisms of action of acupuncture operate at a systematic and general level (no matter what very clever and specific treatment plan we have concocted!).

- Thirdly, the effect of acupuncture will normally tend towards improved overall physiology (no matter where we put the needles or how we manipulate them!). By varying our needling technique we may provoke different short-term effects, mediated through diversions of resources, and which may result in a change in energy transformation and resource apportionment in the body, or its dispersal as heat and motion. But notwithstanding the specific kind of short-term effect provoked, the medium-term one will always tend towards improved physiological balance (provided the organism is not priorly in a very depleted state).

- Fourthly, however artfully we work, the body decides (what, when, and in what time frame).

It follows that attempts on our part to micromanage physiology are superfluous and futile. Such tinkering will be brushed aside by the robust organism like water off a duck's back. But excessively intense or persistent attempts of this kind with a greatly compromised organism carry important risks.

5.4 Super Points

There are acupuncture points that are much more popular than others: recommended time after time in historic and modern textbooks, used more frequently in laboratory and clinical research, and for a much wider range of conditions than other points. Some of them are also those that show more widespread areas of brain activation in functional magnetic resonance imaging studies.

In Chapter 4 I referred to the work of Lee and Chae (2020)[72], Hwang et al. (2020)[73], and Yoo et al. (2022)[74], who separately identified the most widely used points in acupuncture practice. Their findings were strikingly similar. I have summarised them in the table below. Several of these points, notably LI4, LR3 and ST36 are those that produce the most widespread activation of brain regions as demonstrated by fMRI.

---

72 Lee IS, Chae Y. Identification of major traditional acupuncture points for pain control using network analysis. *Acupunct Med*. 2021;39(5):553-554. doi:10.1177/0964528420971309

73 Hwang YC, Lee IS, Ryu Y, Lee YS, Chae Y. Identification of Acupoint Indication from Reverse Inference: Data Mining of Randomized Controlled Clinical Trials. *J Clin Med*. 2020;9(9):3027. Published 2020 Sep 20. doi:10.3390/jcm9093027

74 Yoo Y, Ryu Y, Lee IS, Chae Y. Diachronic analysis of major acupoints used in ancient and current acupuncture treatments: Changes in main acupoints over time. *Integr Med Res*. 2022;11(3):100865. doi:10.1016/j.imr.2022.100865

Major Points	
Upper limbs	HT7, PC6, LI4
Lower limbs	KI3, SP6, LR3, ST36, GB34
Trunk	CV3, CV4, CV6, CV8, CV12, GV20
Head	Yintang

I am particularly interested in those of the above points which are located on the limbs as these (a) usually overlying peripheral sensory nerves, and (b) access longitudinally lying myofascial plains, two media by which I believe the systemic effects of acupuncture are triggered. Based on my reasoning that much disease is in some way stress-induced or stress-aggravated ("stress" in the widest sense), and that the response to acupuncture is basically a stress response, I consider these points to be adaptogenic in nature points because of their systemic regulatory effects, and anti-stress points *par excellence*. They are the major points, super points, that can be used for almost anything treatable!

"Super Points": Adaptogenic Points *Par Excellence*	
Above all	LI4, SP6, LR3, ST36, GB34
Then	HT7, PC6, KI3

To these I would add the following points:

Upper extremity: LU7, TH5, SI3

Lower extremity: KI7 (which I prefer to KI3), BL60, 62

I note that the listed points are all located around the distal joints of the extremities: elbows, wrists, hands, knees, ankles and feet.

Extra-meridian points: *Huatuojiaji*[75], a series of points along the lengths of the paraspinal muscle masses at the level of the intervertebral facet joints can be regarded as adaptogenic if considered as a whole. (The individual points have more compartmentalised significance according to the spinal level involved.) I use an electrically powered percussion device to penetrate the skin with multiple short needles along the posterior midline of the neck and back and the whole length of the erector spinae muscles from occiput to sacrum.

I do this on virtually all of my patients. It can be done with any patient irrespective of their level of vitality, with appropriate variation in both the force of percussion (from extremely light to fairly heavy) and the number of passages (from one to three). I usually use a specially designed electromechanical device for this, but the same can be done with the plum blossom hammer if a lighter touch is required with a sensitive or depleted patient.

The Ear

Shen Men in the ear could also be regarded as a super point judging by its popularity amongst acupuncturists. But I would like to refer the reader to research suggesting that while auricular acupuncture seems to be effective, it does not matter which points are needled (Korelo et al., 2022)[76]. Thus the the external ear may well be regarded s an acupuncture area rather than a collection of discrete points. The sensory innervation of the concha is supplied by the

---

75 Pinyin notation.

76 Korelo RIG, Moreira NB, Miguel BAC, et al. Effects of Auriculotherapy on treatment of women with premenstrual syndrome symptoms: A randomized, placebo-controlled clinical trial. *Complement Ther Med*. 2022;66:102816. doi:10.1016/j.ctim.2022.102816

auricular branch of the vagus[77], and herein may lie its general potency[78].

5.5 Zonal Areas of Influence

I find no reason to believe in meridians as well-defined tracts of energy passage. However, I do believe there are vertically and horizontally arranged zones of influence. I believe these zones can be explained largely on the combined basis of fascial planes and segmental neurology ('tomes'). Below I list the various regions influenced by the vertically aligned zones of the upper (UEX) and lower (LEX) extremities:

Anterior UEX

- Fascial connection: Anterior chest, anterolateral neck, throat.

- Neural connection: C5-T2 (proceeding down lateral side then up medial side of arm).

Posterior UEX

- Fascial connection: Scapular and posterior thoracic region.

- Neural connection: C5-T2 (proceeding down lateral side then up medial side of arm).

---

77 However, other areas of the visible external ear are supplied by either the auricular temporal nerve (CN V3), the lesser occipital nerve or the greater auricular nerve (both cervical plexus, C2-C3) (superioir, middle and inferior thirds respectively).

78 Nevertheless, Haker, Egekvist & Bjerring (2000) found that while acupuncture stimulation of the inferior hemi-concha induced a significant increase in the parasympathetic activity during the stimulation period of 25 min and during the post-stimulation period of 60 min, no significant changes were observed in sympathetic activity, blood pressure or heart rate. Haker E, Egekvist H, Bjerring P. Effect of sensory stimulation (acupuncture) on sympathetic and parasympathetic activities in healthy subjects. *J Auton Nerv Syst.* 2000;79(1):52-59. doi:10.1016/s0165-1838(99)00090-9

Medial UEX

- Fascial connection: Axillary region, lateral middle and lower thorax.
- Neural connection: C8-T2 (from distal to proximal).

Lateral UEX

- Fascial connection: Superior trapezius region, lateral neck.
- Neural connection: C5-C6 (from distal to proximal).

Anterior LEX

- Fascial connection: Anterior abdomen.
- Neural connection: L2-L5 (from proximal to distal).

Posterior LEX

- Fascial connection: Back and posterior neck.
- Neural connection: S1-S2 (from lateral to medial).

Medial LEX

- Fascial connection: Groin, pelvic bowl and abdomen.
- Neural connection: L1-L4 (from proximal to distal).

Lateral LEX

- Fascial connection: Hips, flanks, abdomen.
- Neural connection: L2-S1 (from proximal to distal).

The parts influenced by the fascial network include not only the somatic tissues but also the viscera, glands and vessels enclosed and penetrated by fascia. Similarly, those influenced by the neural connection include not only the somatic tissues but also the viscera, glands and vessels innervated by sympathetic efferents from the same and adjacent spinal levels.

Thus for example, the adrenal glands could be reached via various fascial routes: the posterior and lateral LEX (via the thoracolumbar fascia, quadratus lumborum and the renal fascia), and the anterior LEX (via the psoas muscle and renal fascia). Traditional points such as KI3, KI6 and SP6, situated on the medial leg, which some have proposed may specifically stimulate adrenal function, influence the posterior fascial planes via the soleus / gastrocnemius complex.

Sympathetic innervation to the adrenals is mainly from the T10 to L1 spinal cord segments. So in view of the fact that sensory input to a segment can affect output only a few segments higher and lower, if we used a point on the lower extremity, it would make sense to stimulate dermatomal levels as near to L1 as possible. The upper medial thigh would satisfy this criterion, but in practice we have to balance various criteria. When we factor in the desirability of choosing tender points and points on related deep fascial planes as well, we find ourselves attracted distally, to the lower medial thigh and the medial leg.

5.6 How Specific Can We Get?

As I have said and reiterated, I believe that claims of highly specific treatment (i.e. the treatment of this or that kind of syndrome or energy imbalance by judicious point selection) are overstated. I believe that effective points have a systemic regulatory effect and that this is the same irrespective of the condition treated. Nevertheless, there is a degree of specificity of a topographical nature:

- Specificity based on the vertical and horizontal arrangement of "tomes" and fascial planes, as already explained.

- Specificity based on the quarter of the body treated, as explained in later sections.

- Local specificity. Points local to an injured or diseased part "direct the healing attention" to this part. This is particularly and rapidly evident, for example, in the treatment of myofascial trigger points, but it is certainly not limited to this example.

These possibilities well allow for a sufficient degree of specific treatment. By way of example, let us consider a case of systemic toxicity, manifesting as some kind of widespread inflammatory disease such as arthritis or dermatitis, in which it is also evident that bowel function is compromised (there is chronic constipation and flatulence). Based on our overall assessment of the case, we believe that for the time being, apart from any systemic effect, the best specific "leverage" we might have on the condition of this patient is to improve bowel function. So, in addition to the systemic effect of our treatment, we can "direct some healing attention" more specifically to the bowel, or even just the abdomen.

We may act regionally by needling any tender point in the lower extremities, or any point that, when needled, causes pain or other sensations to radiate centripetally.

We may act via reflex effects through the "tomes": S2 for example (posterior leg) to affect the bowel's parasympathetic supply; T10-12 on the back or abdomen for the sympathetic supply to the ascending and transverse colon; L1 and L2 at the lateral iliac and thigh areas for the sympathetics to the descending colon.

We may act through fascial planes, and here the phrenicocolic ligaments (right and left), connecting the colic flexures to the diaphragm, and Toldt's fascia, which connects it to the posterior abdominal wall, may provide therapeutic avenues. I would be thinking to act via the medial forearm / anterior arm to influence the former, or the anterolateral leg to influence both.

Different things will work for different people, but a good initial approach would be to needle ST36, together with a tender point in the lateral thigh or hip area, plus needling of the trunk in the T10-T12 dermatomes.

Clearly this is a simplification, and meant only to indicate how "healing attention" may be directed. In real life, of course, we would be looking to all influences on bowel function, including digestive secretions and overall functioning, diet, hydration and lifestyle. Should we decide that bowel function is compromised due to insufficient or uncoordinated bile production/delivery, we would "direct the healing attention" accordingly.

Often we will be "aiming" our treatment based on physical signs rather than symptoms: changes in skin texture, humidity, colour and quality, evidence of circulatory changes (heat, cold, swollen veins and capillaries, varices, etc.), changes in subcutaneous texture (toughness, laxness, bogginess, nodules, etc.), hyperaemic skin reactions to palpation, and others. If such signs occur regionally, then we can "direct the healing attention" to the region affected in the same ways as those discussed above.

Here I must remark that I accept that the means by which I have proposed that topographic specificity may be achieved, especially as regards the fascial routes, are highly speculative, but then so are the meridians. I happen to believe my propositions are more realistic speculations!

So, even though I say that the main effect of treatment is systemic, I still allow that there is ample opportunity for topographical specificity. Nevertheless, I must reiterate a point I have made elsewhere, about the pitfalls of attempts at micromanagement.

The patient's organism has much more unconscious intelligence than your or my conscious mind! It has its own therapeutic plan, and while we can facilitate the expression of that plan, we cannot command the precise character or time frame of its evolution. The more complex our clinical reasoning becomes, the more we expose ourselves to error, and the less, not the more, control we have. The more we believe we can manipulate the patient's energy precisely by our own design, the more deluded we have become!

What if it were possible to precisely target acupuncture effect to internal or systemic diseases by needling peripheral points? Would this be an advisable thing to do? Would it improve outcomes?

I begin with the premise that acupuncture treatment is neither specifically "tonifying" nor specifically "dispersing" (or whichever other words one might like to use) but normalising. There may be an initial excitation or inhibition but when that subsides homeostasis will settle at a new normal.

Secondly, hyper or hypofunction in a tissue, organ or system is often driven by physiological demands elsewhere. In this case, attempts to influence it directly will be futile. Further, in a chronic context, even though the dysfunction were once primary, reciprocal adaptations in other parts soon become so well integrated that primacy becomes irrelevant. The result of direct attention to one element of the system will be equally futile. It follows the acute setting is the only one in which directly targeting the dysfunctional tissue, organ or system might be appropriate.

While I accept that Chinese medicine may make attempts to address the whole system via the five-phase model, I am of the opinion that the impression of understanding gained through its manipulation are illusory. I feel that in reality we do not possess sufficient knowledge truly to know exactly how and why the body's intelligence has set up its internal economy and dynamics in the way it has. So targeting this or that organ or system is like shooting in the dark. We think we know what we are doing but we really don't that much.

We need a conceptually simple therapeutic system which is tolerant of ignorance and error, and a general treatment which trusts the body's own intelligence rather than a suffocating and futile exercise in micromanagement. We need only to target the one system we know we can most directly influence, the nervous system.

5.7 Treatment Heuristics

Although acupuncture produces a general and systemic response and this is the most valuable thing when dealing with non-musculoskeletal disorders, we can still benefit from some guiding principles to focus the healing attention, as well as empirical pragmatism where those principles fail or do not reach[79]. It is certainly the case that different subjects will respond to different points at different times, so guiding principles help us better to manage this. I have stated my feeling that the guiding principles of traditionalists are over-cooked, dogmatic, and often illusory. I propose a different, simpler set

Now at this point I think we can introduce some rules of thumb and some strategies which I have found to be successful in practice:

1. Needling any part of the body can potentially produce systemic effects.

2. Needling the upper limbs can potentially achieve greater

---

79 The conflict, or better, dynamic, between principles and pragmatism is not a uniquely modern or Western dilemma. It exists deep within the acupuncture taught in modern China, that practice having being artificially standardised to one overarching abstract rationale but somewhat paradoxically often falling back on a down-to-earth empiricism unburdened by theoretical machinations (i.e. points recommended for this or that symptom).

effects in the upper body (let us say, as a rough rule, the parts of the body above the diaphragm).

3. Needling the lower limbs can potentially achieve greater effects in the lower body (let us say, as a rough rule, the parts of the body below the mid-abdominal region).

4. To achieve effects in the upper abdominal region, needle both upper and lower limbs.

5. Needling one side of the body can potentially achieve greater effects on the same side of the body. This combined with numbers 2 and 3 above means that needling any limb "directs the healing attention" regionally to that quarter of the body.

6. Combine needling according to vertical organisation with that according to horizontal organisation. By doing so, we are using a crude grid and coordinate system to focus treatment effects insofar as that is possible. For instance, stimulation of the medial leg combined with stimulation in the lower thoracic / upper lumbar and/or sacral regions may be expected to influence the intra-pelvic organs.

7. Points below the knee and elbow are especially useful, possibly because these parts are more sensitive than other areas.

8. Choose one or both of these strategies (if both can be achieved with a single needle, so much the better!):

    a. Needle the "tome" of the spinal nerve nearest the sympathetic ganglia that innervates the organs one wishes to influence.

    b. Needle a fascial plane continuous by an uncomplicated route with the target area.

9. Choose preferably points to needle any which are tender and/or, when pressed or needled cause pain to radiate

towards the area one wishes to influence.

10. Otherwise (or at the same time) choose points that are much used traditionally for a wide range of purposes.

11. If 7, 8 and 9 can be combined all in one point, this is the best strategy of all!

12. Be sparing in needle use! As a general rule, for a systemic effect, try not to use more than one needle per limb, and not more than two on the trunk, neck, head and face.

13. To direct attention strongly to a local and superficial musculoskeletal complaint (e.g. tendonitis), more needles and/or more intense stimulation may be used in the affected area.

14. Trigger and tender points: Stimulate a maximum of four points at a time.

15. If one can obtain in the patient, by needle manipulation, a feeling of heaviness or pressure, dull aching or cramp-like pain, numbness or tingling (around the needle if local to an affected area, towards the affected area, or proximally towards the body for a systemic effect) - traditionally known as *deqi* - this is a good predictor of a beneficial outcome.

16. Strength of stimulation: Stimulation should be the weakest that will effectively produce a healing response. This will vary according to the vitality and reactivity of the patient. Begin with moderately weak stimulation to assess the response before adjusting the treatment at subsequent sessions.

5.8 Treatment Criteria and Strategies

5.8.1 Symptomatic Treatment

The symptomatic approach, if left at that, is not always the best we can do for our patients. However, it may be all they want. While fully informing our patients, we must prioritise their wishes and expectations in the planning and execution of our treatment plan. In actual practice, I rarely find any conflict. My view is that in acute conditions, symptomatic treatment is the priority, while in chronic contexts, systemic treatment works best. What does it mean to treat symptomatically? To put it simply but quite accurately, it is when we treat locally, needle where it hurts, apply warmth where its cold, cool where its hot. And systemically? This requires a model, even a rudimentary one, about how the body works in health and illness; the predisposition to look for connections and the effort to search for signs.

5.8.2 Mode/Stage of the General Adaptation Syndrome

In 1936 Hans Selye coined the word stress to describe "a non-specific response of the body to any demand for change"[80]. This non-specific response was further described by Selye as the General Adaptation Syndrome (GAS). The GAS model proposes three stages in the physiological stress response: Alarm, Resistance and Exhaustion. I prefer to use the term "modes" rather than stages because there is no inevitability that under stress an organism will pass linearly through them starting from Alarm and proceeding to Resistance then Exhaustion to the bitter end.

Treatment on the basis of the mode of the GAS is, for all practical

---

80 Selye H. A Syndrome produced by Diverse Nocuous Agents. *Nature.* 1936;138:32. https://doi.org/10.1038/138032a0

purposes, the same as saying treatment on the basis of the phase of illness: acute, chronic, advanced chronic.

GAS mode 1 (alarm physiology, acute symptoms)

Symptomatic treatment. But we should be aware that many acute stage symptoms are actually repeat exacerbations of underlying chronic dysfunction, in which case the benefit of symptomatic treatment will be limited in time unless backed up by systemic treatment.

GAS mode 2 (resistance physiology, chronic symptoms)

Systemic treatment. This will usually involve, literally, all four corners of the body. We are more concerned with how this patient will be in two years time than how they will feel tomorrow. It will not be a straightforward journey, the line on the graph will not be smooth, straight, always upwards. There will be ups and downs to manage, but hopefully after 18 months the patient will be noticeably better than (s)he was before.

GAS mode 3 (exhaustion physiology, chronic pathology)

Treatment and management will be geared towards, (1) conservation of energy and other resources; (2) good nutrition; (3) support of the body's main physiological systems, particularly digestion, elimination, circulation and respiration; (4) autonomic regulation. It will not be about "stimulating the adrenals", but about providing them with a nourishing and non-toxic environment. We have to let tired organs rest. Treatment will be slow and gentle, as will improvement.

5.8.3 Vitality Level

Patients obviously vary in their responsiveness to stimuli in general, and needling in particular. This responsiveness is organism-wide, involving the cognitive and emotional appreciation of the therapeutic act as well as the bodily one. Some patients require vigorous needling to produce any worthwhile response. Others would be left depleted by such an approach. Patients with low vitality are best treated with few, fine needles, without much needle manipulation, in relatively short sessions. Over-stimulation may produce an unpleasant acute reaction and/or further depletion of vital resources.

5.8.4 Constitution

French acupuncturist Yves Requena has described his approach to treatment based on six types of terrain: the *Tai Yang, Shao Yang, Yang Ming, Tai Yin, Shao Yin, Jue Yin*[81]. Many of you will recognise these (or alternative transliterations of them) as the six major pathways through the body comprising of coupled meridians. Each combines one meridian from the lower half of the body with one from the upper half. Requena postulated that each of us tends to be influenced by one of these pathways more than the others, and that this influence determines our physiological and psychological characteristics in illness and in health. Perhaps paradoxically, in view of my stated stance on meridians (they do not exist as such) I have found these categorisations to be useful in that they do seem to have the real power to predict where in the body, under stress, symptoms will first and most frequently appear - where the weakest links, so to speak, are likely to be. The apparent contradiction I make is resolved when I say that I consider that these categories point to functional relations rather than physical meridians. Thus, if a patient is quite clearly classifiable into one of those six categories over and

---

81 Requena Y. *Terrains et Pathologie en Acupuncture*. Maloine; 1980.

above the others, we may choose areas that are functionally related (by fascial planes or "tomal" level) to the organs comprising their "weakest links", in order to explore for tender points or otherwise deliver treatment.

Influenced by Requena, I developed my own, (again, highly speculative!) stress-based understanding of human constitution in a series of four articles published in the International Journal of Alternative and Complementary Medicine in 1995 and 1996. In the Appendix I summarise the content of these articles. My thesis is that pathogenesis may be described very well by reference to two variables: the activity of a physiological function (say, SNS activity), and the tension in the system. The basic paths to ill health allowed by this description mirror fairly closely those suggested by Requena's six types of terrain. Fundamentally, how we get ill depends on (a) our tendency to heightened or reduced activity of the major control systems (CNS, ANS, endocrine, immune), and (b) our innate vitality level.

This model proposes two fundamental attributes of any pathological process, responsiveness to stimuli, and tension in the system. It allows us to predict an individual's response to acupuncture to the extent that we can recognise the type of the individual according to this classificatory scheme. We must be mindful of both these variables when planning and executing treatment. Furthermore, considering these variables in our patient is an essential step in forming a reasoned prognosis.

5.8.5 Zonal Areas of Influence

In *Reinventing Acupuncture* Felix Mann[82] described how he found the four limbs to provide therapeutic avenues to the corresponding

---

82 Mann F. *Reinventing Acupuncture. A New Concept of an Ancient Medicine.* 2nd edition. Butterworth-Heinemann; 2000.

four corners of the body. That is, for example, if one is attempting to treat symptoms arising from the left iliac fossa area, one would treat suitable points on the left leg; if one has to treat a right-sided neck or thoracic pain, the right arm would be treated[83]. (Interestingly, though, his favourite point was LR3, not only for "livery" symptoms or lower body symptoms, but also, for instance, for headaches. Well, we all have our favourites, and they do tend to be points that have been used much throughout the ages, which as I have said probably indicates a general adaptogenic capability.) Another example, SP9, on the medial tibial condyle, is good for all conditions affecting the inner and medial knee, as well as pelvic conditions. The examples are numerous. In my experience, Mann's idea of regional and zonal tropisms is correct and well-worth exploitation.

Wrist and ankle acupuncture is a modern style of acupuncture developed by Zhang Xinshu[84] which divides the body into six vertically arranged regions. Needling one of twelve specific points at the wrist or ankle is said to influence pathology in the corresponding vertical region, above or below the diaphragm respectively. Essentially it is similar to what I propose so far as specificity is concerned, although I find the six regions to be too categorically defined and the choice of only twelve defined points very limiting.

5.8.6 Tenderness as a Criterion for Needling

I believe tenderness to be an obvious, reliable and valid method of selecting points for acupuncture treatment. This is because tenderness directly indicates those tissues that are involved in the body's integrated response to challenge or insult.

Topographic features such as depressions or furrows in the superficial tissues of the body indicate places where we may readily

---

83 The situation with the head and face may be somewhat more complex, given that, with the exception of CN2, 4, 7 and 12, the cranial nerves do not decussate.
84 Xinshu Z. Wrist and Ankle Acupuncture Therapy. *JCM*. 1991;7:5-14.

connect with fascial planes and junctions. Tender points (*ah-shi / ah shi / ashi* points in TCM) are often found in these places. Often, running one's fingers lightly along furrows between muscle bundles or tendons, or along borders where muscle meets bone, one is called to linger at certain points. It may be that a subtle depression is detected, or there is some minute swelling or change in skin drag or tissue quality. Almost invariably these points are tender.

My preferred method is to seek out tenderness in the areas most suggested by the characteristics of the case, then to needle deeply enough to reach the muscle or fascial tissue in which the tenderness is located.

There are many maps of tender points and tender areas which may appear in the body's superficial tissues. The following are some of the reference points I like to use for palpation:

- The inter-metacarpal and inter-metatarsal spaces.

- The depressions around joints.

- In the forearms the furrows between tendons or muscles, and the areas near the humeral epicondyles.

- Around the shoulders, the supra- and infraspinatus, subacromial and deltoid areas, the coracoid process.

- In the legs (below the knee) the depressions, furrows and junctions between muscle, tendon, fascia and bone, the medial tibial condyle.

- Around the hips, just inferior to the iliac crests, the supra and posterior trocanteric areas

- With respect to any muscle, the musculotendinous junctions.

- With respect to the back, the interspinous ligaments, the paraspinal fossae, the posterior sacroiliac ligaments.

- With respect to the posterior neck, the muscle mass over the articular pillars.

- With respect to the head and face: along the inferior occiput from the midline to the mastoid process of the temporal bone, the parietal origins of the temporalis muscle, the masseter muscle body.

- With respect to the abdomen: scanning palpation for superficial tissue quality and skin-rolling for tenderness, deeper palpation for areas of tension and tenderness in the muscular wall.

- With respect to the anterior rib cage, the anterior end of intercostal spaces, especially those adjacent to the sternum. One must remain very aware of the potential for excessively deep needling here to cause pneumothorax.

5.8.7 Treatment Based on the Pulses

These will possibly be my most controversial paragraphs. Traditionalists may scorn and deride me as an ignoramus. Scientific rationalists may scorn and deride me as a purveyor of mumbo-jumbo. However, I take heart in this: there is no way that either can prove me wrong!

First, an unassailable fact. "Traditional" taking of the radial pulse is described differently in different classic texts, and has been practised differently by different practitioners from different cultures (Chinese, Japanese, etc.) and eras. The most obvious difference is in the positions ascribed to different physiological systems/functions. Yet there is no evidence to suggest that acupuncture is more or less effective when practised by pulse-takers of different persuasions. I take it that there is a lot of unverifiable theory and dogma surrounding what is fundamentally an intuitive clinical method.

I go further. My contention is that traditional pulse-taking is an act of dowsing. I am of the opinion that direct (if you like "extra-sensory") knowledge about the nature of things is a common occurrence. Moreover, it is a phenomenon that can be trained, that is, it can be performed at will in an organised way under the right conditions and with enough practice.

The right conditions are mental concentration and intent. It is helpful to have a catalyst, and this function is provided by a meaningful ritual. In our case the meaningful ritual is the taking of the pulse. When I take your pulse and I focus with concentration on what I have taken to be such and such a physiological system, in my mind there is a question: What is happening with this physiological system? And lo, I obtain my answer.

We need to recognise that it is not an objective examination. Since it has an important subjective element, there is considerable potential for the intrusion of fantasy and imagination. In such a context, the more complex our model, the more numerous the pitfalls. So let us not forget also that any interpretation based on pulse-taking must be backed up by other observations from general clinical examination. Happily, my approach to acupuncture requires a much less elaborate theoretical framework than the version of tradition that is today taught as standard.

So I accept that traditional pulse-taking may have diagnostic validity (if not inter-practitioner reliability). But how much of that information is going to be useful to me in treatment considering the theoretical basis that I have described in this text? What useful questions can I ask the pulse? Because my theoretical base is simple, I can dispense with some aspects of the mechanics of pulse-taking, many of the traditionally described nuances of pulse quality, and the bulk of diagnostic interpretations. Most important of all are questions about overall vitality, energy in the system, tension in the system, the rate at which physiology proceeds (hyper-, hypo-, and normo-) and reactivity (responsiveness). These will tell me about how to needle. And actually these most important, basic questions depend less on my ability as a dowser, because the answers are given by real physical qualities of the pulse (albeit subjectively appreciated).

Vitality

A vital pulse is regular, firm and and elastic. It is easily palpable and does not disappear when moderate pressure is exerted. A pulse that aggressively punches at the fingers means vitality is strained. A weak, sluggish pulse, lacks vitality.

Energy level and tension

Bounding, overflowing, finger-punching, hammering pulses mean there is excess energy in a tense system. The system is highly-strung. Weak, sluggish pulses denote lack of energy in loosely strung system.

Sometimes one finds the qualities "tightness" and "weakness" together. Here we have a manifestation of tension in a system lacking in energy. Or we may perceive an overflowing pulse without much "oomph", interpretable as an energetic system working at low tension.

Rate and reactivity (responsiveness)

If the pulse is fast the system is accelerated, if slow it is damped down. If its frequency fluctuates greatly in response to mild challenge (e.g. the very act of pulse taking, the insertion of an acupuncture needle), the system is excitable, highly reactive.

5.8.8 Autonomic Balance

I have stated previously that I believe autonomic balance to be at the heart of pathophysiology. Sympathetic activity is immediately responsive to changes in environmental variables. There lies our point of leverage. Anyone who has experience of working manually on the body will have noticed the gurgling sounds coming from the intestines of the patient either when some release is achieved (particularly of the cervical vertebrae) or when the patient is becoming nicely relaxed. This is due to a reduction of sympathetic tone. In the following hours and days sympathetic tone and reactivity often tend to reset to new, more normally physiological levels. A similar resetting occurs after acupuncture treatment. As stated previously, this is not so much the specific effect of specific points, but a general, systemic effect of both the needling and the therapeutic context.

But how can we gauge sympathetic function? Firstly, is the sympathetic highly excitable? Secondly, is there a high level of tension in the system? Then, a further question suggests itself: What is the utility of this information?

Is the Sympathetic Highly Excitable?

Tell-tale signs are found in symptoms, behaviour and clinical responses.

Symptoms: Palpitations, reactive hypertension (especially systolic), bouts of sweating, suddenly feeling hot or cold, hot flushes, "butterflies in the stomach", bouts of vertigo or nausea, hyperventilation, symptoms reactive to stressful events.

Behaviour: Unease, nervousness, easily alarmed or startled, over-emotional reactions.

Clinical responses: Generalised hyperreflexia, extensive hyperaemic skin reactions to palpation, distress disproportionate to objective findings, unexpectedly strong reactions to treatment.

Is There a High Level of Tension in the System?

A high level of tension in the system denotes a move to chronicity, and a blunting of precise, context-dependent control of physiological functions. Elsewhere I have called this condition "stiffness". Some of its most common symptoms are generalised anxiety, chronic shoulder, neck and jaw pain, bruxism, tension headaches, arterial hypertension (systolic and diastolic), visceral spasms, chronic gastrointestinal dysfunction, gastro-oesophageal reflux, irritable bowel syndrome, sleep disturbance, irritability, reduced motivation, compensatory behaviours (excessive smoking, drinking), social avoidance.

What is the Utility of the Information?

This may seem an odd question. The whole thesis of this book is that much pathophysiology is stress-based. Sympathetic activation is a stress response. So, of course it should be useful to determine its characteristics, shouldn't it? On the other hand I have said that acupuncture treatment does not have to be specific and that responses to it are largely systemic and normalising, whatever the characteristics of the pathology or dysfunction, so it shouldn't matter, should it?

My answer is this: the value of this information is not in that it tells us necessarily *where* to needle, but in that it can give us guidance on *how* to needle. A highly excitable system will respond to brief, gentle, superficial needling but will react negatively in the short term to over-treatment, to the patient's distress.

Raised "tension", for all intents and purposes, corresponds to resistance physiology, with chronic autonomic activation. High levels of tension often go hand in hand with reduced responsiveness ("stiffness"), so longer, more intense, deeper needling is required to provoke a regulatory response.

On the other hand, low tension often signifies low vitality. Some people simply lack the reserves to respond very much and strong treatment will exhaust them. Stimulation needs to be lighter and more frequent, but not too frequent. It is a subtle balancing act.

5.8.9 Needling Variables

There are three main variables, needle depth, needle manipulation, and treatment time, discussed below. In all cases we have to take into account the overall vitality, systemic tension, and reactivity of our patient. As a rule, stimulation should be the weakest that will effectively produce a healing response. The safe thing to do is to begin with moderately weak stimulation to assess the response before adjusting the treatment at subsequent sessions. It is worth planning more sessions rather than less in order to allow for this effort of calibration. For local areas of pain or inflammation that are directly accessibly, stronger needling will often produce the best effect (by the principle of counter-irritation).

Needle Depth

This depends on the structures one desires to reach (skin, muscle, fascia, periosteum, ligament) and the vitality level of the patient. In most cases of general treatment I wish the needles in the limbs to reach muscle and/or deep fascial tissue. However in very depleted or highly reactive subjects I may wish to puncture shallowly, just penetrating the skin and subcutaneous tissue.

Needle Manipulation

- Trigger points and superficial needling need no needle manipulation.
- In my opinion any "tonifying" or "inhibitory" effects depend

neither on the material of which the needle is made nor on the direction of needle manipulation, but only on the duration and vigour of manipulation. It is important to realise that such effects are short-term. This may be important in acute scenarios, but it is irrelevant in chronic ones (as the overall medium to long-term effect of needling is adaptogenic), except insofar as very weak subjects verging on exhaustion physiology may be "tipped over the edge" by over-vigorous or extended treatment.

- To achieve a needling sensation of dull pain, heaviness, pressure, numbness, tingling, or pain radiation, needle manipulation is required. Usually persistent rotation of the needle is sufficient, but sometimes repetitive quick partial withdrawal and thrust bring about the sensation more rapidly. Rotation does not have to be in any determined direction.

Treatment time

- Trigger points require no more than 5 minutes.

- Very weak patients and very reactive patients require no more than 5 minutes.

- Stronger or less sensitive patients may benefit from up to half an hour.

- Patients often relax during acupuncture treatment. This is beneficial. Up to half an hour may be allowed if this is the priority. More is unnecessary and the patient may become fidgety. Even relaxation has its time.

5.8.10 Management Variables

Treatment frequency and time scale are widely variable. Frequency can vary from once a day to once every few months. The time scale can be one week or forever. Quite apart from organisational considerations, they depend on:

1. The patient's vitality.

2. The nature of the patient's condition.

3. The stage of the patient's condition (acute, subacute, chronic, advanced).

4. The mode of the GAS.

5. The constitution of the patient.

6. The patient's goals and expectations.

How to provide a simple, concise, rule-of-thumb exposition of all this? Here are some ideas:

Frequent treatment is given when little and often is the best strategy, that is, in very acute conditions and very weak patients. One has to bear in mind however that "often" can also be too often!

Less frequent treatment is given when the patient is highly reactive or their condition more chronic.

Infrequent but regular treatment is given for maintenance.

Brief courses of treatment may be all that is necessary for recent, uncomplicated cases.

Extended courses of treatment will be required in chronic conditions or with particularly unresponsive patients.

In my practice, the most typical scenario is of a moderately chronic condition that will require up to 10 weekly treatments initially, with follow ups at one and three months. Further follow-ups / maintenance to be decided according to the patient's progress.

It is a fact of life that cost considerations and acceptability to the patient of the treatment plan make Western practice different from Chinese practice, in which the same moderately chronic patient described in the last paragraph may be treated three times a week for twenty weeks

5.8.11 Achieving the Right Total Environment

Many years ago as an undergraduate biology student I went to an extracurricular lecture given by a practising acupuncturist who said something I have always remembered, and that was that to stay healthy we must be kind to our meridians. Allowing for the poetic use of metaphor, that is what this section is about.

There are certain basic conditions of one's total environment that need to be satisfied in order to create a context which promotes vitality and health rather than detracting from them. The benefit of any kind of treatment will be limited, to an extent which may even be total, unless the patient's total environment is conducive to healing. And a healthy environment is the only true healer.

One's total environment includes the physical, chemical, biological, social and aesthetic environments. It also includes our inner environment: physical, chemical, cognitive, emotional. Such things, for example, as negative habits of thought, influence our total environment.

While the precise conditions for health are different for each of us, its basic components are the same: clean air, right food, clean water, right exercise, right rest and relaxation, right sleep, right social interaction, right physical surroundings, right challenges, motivations, outlook, and so on.

The word "right" in the above list means appropriate in kind and amount. Clearly what is "right" for one person is not "right" for another. What is a stimulating challenge for one person may be a tiresome burden for another, and the difference is accounted for not only by everything else in the person's total environment, but also by their constitutional potential and predilections.

Thus, encouraging and facilitating the creation of a healthful total environment is fundamental to any form of real healing. To this end one or both of two basic strategies may be employed, according to the person's condition and needs at the time. One can reduce the negative load in areas or contexts in which it is proving too much. In the context of diet this could mean eliminating foods to which a person is intolerant, for instance. In the context of overwork, it could mean allowing oneself to avoid certain duties. Secondly, one can develop the resources necessary to more easily cope with those aspects of life that are burdensome. In the same two contexts: improving gut integrity and function; improving organisational skills, for instance.

This kind of thing has been called stress management. But it is really life management! Many, many people become ill because they are not coping well with life. I have written about this in my book, "Stress: Survive and Thrive" (Avicenna, 2016).

5.9 A Typical Treatment

In what follows I do not want the reader to think I am trying to "teach grandmother to suck eggs" or that I believe this is the only way of doing it. I have more respect and humility than that. In all cases you should understand that I am simply describing what I personally do in practice.

With systemic treatment, at the first session I nearly always needle two "super points" bilaterally: ST36 and LI4. I return to these two points at alternate sessions. In the intervening sessions, if tension and/or energy is low, I more often favour points on the medial aspects of the lower and anteromedial aspects of the upper extremities. Conversely, if tension/energy is high, I favour the lateral and posterolateral aspects respectively. The parts treated usually include points below the elbow and knee[85]. Both upper and lower limbs are treated bilaterally. Usually 4 to 8 needles are used for this treatment.

On the second and thereafter every second treatment I use my mechanical "plum blossom" hammer all down the midline and paraspinal muscle masses from the occiput to the fifth sacral segment. I do this at the beginning of the treatment to "prime" the system, as it were.

I treat the ear, for a non-specific effect. This will include one or two two needles in each ear, Shen Men on one side or the other (I alternate), the others depending on any particular areas to be reached according to the established inverted-foetus model. I do this not because I believe in the model, but because I am superstitious and because it provides a convenient "random point generator" to arrange needles in different areas of the ear without my having to deliberately choose random points!

It may be that I do wish to attempt to be more specific in treatment, and then I may emphasise certain areas in treatment to a greater or lesser extent. This often depends upon whether the symptoms are acute (more specific, locally focused treatment) or chronic (more systemic, general treatment). In what cases may I attempt this more specific treatment? Firstly, the symptoms may be located in a specific part of the body. Secondly, there may be clinical signs of local pathology or dysfunction. Thirdly, I may judge that the best leverage I have right now on this person's overall condition is to

---

85 These are aspects of treatment which were ingrained in me by my acupuncture training (or my understanding of it) and they have served me well. I have no way of knowing whether or not they are really more valid practices than doing otherwise, and I will freely admit that I have kept to them more out of superstition than cold reason. Maybe to deviate more from this scheme and "see what happens" will be the next step in the development of the ideas presented in this book.

attempt to "direct the healing attention to some specific part or system of the body". This commonly happens when the patient complains of an array of symptoms, but one particular symptom is taking a predominant toll on the person's physical and psychological resources, such that its diminution would initiate a general improvement in their health. Or I may judge that an improvement in a particular function, for example digestion, may initiate such a general improvement. In that case I might choose to direct the healing attention to that area of digestive physiology where dysfunction were evident. Such added specificity may be achieved by various means:

1. Needling trigger points.

2. Needling tender points local to symptomatic areas.

3. More aggressive treatment to local areas of pain or inflammation. This could involve a cluster of needles, the plum blossom hammer, or bleeding.

4. Needling a specific limb corresponding to the quarter of the body where symptoms or pathology are located.

5. Treating points on the trunk in combination with those on the limbs, according to a sort of grid and coordinate system, following the notions of vertical and horizontal organisation already outlined.

I have already described my criteria for good points to puncture. Briefly again, they are these:

1. Tenderness.

2. Radiation of pain to symptomatic area.

3. Dermatomal, myotomal or sclerotomal significance.

4. Fascial significance.

5. "Super points".

6. Ease of achievement of a local feeling of heaviness or

pressure, dull aching or cramp-like pain, numbness or tingling on needle manipulation.

If one can combine several of these criteria with a single needle then it is a really good point to treat! In total, for systemic treatment, I usually use between 4 and 8 needles on the limbs. More may be used, including needles on the abdomen/thorax/neck/head/face, when more local or specific treatment is required.

Summary and Conclusion

My contentions throughout this book have been that:

- As a whole the theoretical basis of traditional Chinese acupuncture is over-developed and largely superfluous.

- A simpler theoretical basis for practice is likely to be more efficient and at least as effective.

- Stress, conceived as "any tension generated by our interaction with the outside world" is a major causative, maintaining or aggravating factor in many conditions of ill-health.

- The therapeutic response to acupuncture is a stress response with systemic, regional and local components.

- Even the regional and local components of this response are mediated, modulated, and coordinated centrally.

- In the treatment of chronic conditions, the system-wide response is the most important.

- Tenderness, historic frequency of use, and traditional versatility, are excellent means for selecting points for treatment.

- Fascial planes, "tomes", and regional location provide important means of attempting to "direct healing attention" more specifically.

- But highly specific responses to specific point combinations are likely to be largely illusory.

- Acupuncture is fundamentally adaptogenic.

These are some of my conclusions after twenty-eight years of clinical practice. However, as I am always very aware of the need to be humble, faced with the wonder of life and the mysteries of the universe, let me say this... I may be wrong.

Appendix: A Stress-Based Understanding of Constitution

This is a brief summary and adaptation of three articles written by me and published in the International Journal of Alternative and Complementary Medicine in 1995 and 1996[86][87][88].

The component concepts of my model are: a systems view, allostasis, physiological elasticity, functional uncoupling, relationship with Selye's GAS, a bidimensional description of pathology, archetypal paths to ill health.

A Systems View

The individual human being may be seen as a subsystem within a series of ever more encompassing wider worlds, while being in turn composed of its own series and hierarchies of subsystems working together with extraordinary, intricate complexity. Thus, in order to talk or think about the human being with any degree of reality, one must cultivate the capacity and inclination to zoom into and zoom out from seeing the one and the many, the general and the particular, with agility and over a wide range. But in order to interact with the human being in a pragmatic way (for instance therapeutically), we must be humble: we cannot micromanage such complexity (especially with all its "known and unknown unknowns"), so we must simplify in useful ways. The ancients resolved this by thinking in terms of dichotomous pairs such as *Yin-Yang*, hot-cold, humid-dry, which remarkably, are still pragmatically useful to this day.

---

86   Hale RD. Disease and stress. *IJACM*. 1995;June:19-23.
87   Hale RD. Adapting to disaster. *IJACM*. 1995;November:8-10,31.
88   Hale RD. Measuring the individual. *IJACM*. 1996;August:9-12.

Allostasis

While homeostasis ensures that physiological parameters are kept within healthy limits in the short term, allostasis does the same in the long term. Homeostasis provides a range of responses over a range of stimulus levels. Allostasis involves a wholesale shift in the relationship of response to stimulus. Such long-term adaptation in any one physiological parameter will require widespread compensatory adaptations in others. There is a limit to which such a shift can occur before the internal economy of the body begins to become less energy-efficient and more costly in terms of resources. There is also a limit beyond which no further adaptation would be achievable or compatible with life.

I envisage two basic mechanisms involved in an allostatic shift in response to environmental demands. Firstly, there may be a change in threshold stimulus. That is, the minimum stimulus required to elicit a response. I would associate these changes with the early stages of resistance physiology. Secondly (and secondarily), there may be a change in gain: the degree of response to a given change in stimulus. I associate these changes with the later stages of resistance physiology.

Physiological Elasticity

One way of looking at disease is in terms of an organism's failure to respond appropriately to environmental changes which lie within the ordinary range. I find that a useful way to conceptualise the changes that may occur is to use the metaphors elasticity, stiffness, and plasticity (or laxity).

In normal physiology, homeostasis displays the organism's elasticity. Some stimulus swings a physiological parameter away from its normal baseline, and mechanisms are activated which swing it back again. It may then overshoot slightly the other way, briefly, before the opposite mechanisms bring it back again. This may happen over several cycles of ever diminishing waves, just like a bouncing rubber ball.

When wholesale shifts occur in stimulus-response behaviour, at some point physiological tolerance is diminished. Responses may become deadened or they may become exaggerated. In the one case elasticity has given way to stiffness (rigidity), in the other to plasticity/laxity. Stiffness means relative unresponsiveness to changes in the immediate (internal) or wider (external) environment. Plasticity/laxity, on the other hand, signifies loss of control over the internal environment, which is subject to wider fluctuations depending on external circumstances, or being "blown away by the merest breeze", to use a metaphor.

Deviation from normal physiology may be towards states of heightened or lessened activity, towards a less flexible range of responses (stiffness), or a less controlled range (plasticity/laxity). Elasticity, rigidity and plasticity/laxity manifest themselves physically, physiologically, behaviourally and emotionally.

Functional Uncoupling

This is a term I coined to describe the uncoupling of one function from another, normally dependent function. Functional uncoupling is synonymous with "dys-integration" of control systems, which typically involve negative feedback loops. One example of this is the development of insulin resistance in pre-diabetic states. Tissues become progressively less responsive to insulin, and therefore blood sugar control is compromised. In this example sugar metabolism is uncoupled from insulin secretion and energy management is uncoupled from blood sugar availability. Functional uncoupling is associated with chronic pathology, and the second (and secondary) type of allostatic adaptation, that is, a change in the degree of response to a given change in stimulus.

Relationship with Selye's GAS

These concepts are easily related to Selye's General Adaptation Syndrome.

Stage/Mode 1 of the GAS relates to normal, physiological responses following initial exposure to a stressor of any kind, including injury or infection, for example. This is normally self-limiting in the healthy individual. (Incidentally, this observation actually throws into question our whole notion of pathology: are acute symptoms necessarily "pathological"?) Stage/Mode 1 displays elasticity.

Stage/Mode 2 of the GAS necessarily involves allostatic adaptations to longer term stress. Initially this means changes in stimulus thresholds for physiological responses. Later, it means wholesale changes in the relationship of responses to stimuli. This is when functional uncoupling begins. Stage/Mode 2 displays stiffness. This may have a functional role, in reducing the risk of physiological parameters reaching dangerous levels. However, its benefits become increasingly outweighed by its disadvantages, firstly because it is resource inefficient, secondly because specific sub-systems function with less precise reference to the requirements of other sub-systems within the wider system.

Stage/Mode 3 is when the "dys-integration" of the network of control systems has damaged the organism to such an extent that it no longer possesses the means easily to recover. The organism is "exhausted" of energy and other resources. At an advanced stage, positive feedback loops may begin to replace negative feedback, leading to ever increasing disorganisation. Stage/Mode 3 displays plasticity/laxity.

A Bidimensional Description of Pathology

Let us take a gradient in a physiological variable. It may be postural, metabolic, immunological, endocrine, biochemical, haematological, etc. Any variable we choose will be subject to multiple influences and will in turn influence multiple dependent variables. One primary influence is the autonomic nervous system (ANS). The latter, in fact, in the hierarchy of functions, is one of the highest. Indeed, we shall take this as our example, while allowing that the same general phenomena apply to all physiological variables. The ANS is a convenient example because it consists of identifiable complementary parts (sympathetic and parasympathetic), representing opposite physiological tendencies, and that is essential for our model. However, we could do this with any variable. For blood sugar, although it is not in itself constituted by two components in the same way, we can nevertheless speak about two opposing and complementary homoeostatic tendencies: a tendency to raise and a tendency to reduce blood sugar. The essential point is, physiology is the vital balance between opposite tendencies (*Yin* and *Yang*).

Now, in this context, dysfunction may be of four types:

1. Dominance of one tendency. In our example of the ANS, this could be:

    a. Sympathetic dominance (raised sympathetic tone).

    b. Parasympathetic dominance (reduced sympathetic tone).

2. Global hyperfunction (raised tone of both sympathetic and parasympathetic branches). I envisage that this most commonly comes about through a primary chronic increase in sympathetic activity. Parasympathetic up-regulation is an attempt to compensate for this. Some balance is restored but in a highly tense, energetic system. Precise moment-to-moment control is compromised. The system is less able to

respond appropriately and with sufficient elasticity. It is "stiff", and functional uncoupling begins. To quote Chappell (1984), "If there is an excess of tension in the system, the ability to reciprocate is lost and the system is unable to resonate."[89]

3. Global hypofunction (reduced tone of both sympathetic and parasympathetic branches). Homoeostasis is failing, vitality is deficient. Sympathetic and parasympathetic activation interact only loosely. They are no longer matched either to each other or to physiological needs. The organism is at the mercy of external forces. It is "plastic".

Let us now consider the physiological variable "sympathetic activity" and plot it on a horizontal axis. This axis represents our functional dimension. On the left we have values representing relative hypofunction, and on the right relative hyperfunction. We shall draw another axis, the vertical one, which intersects the horizontal axis at its centre. The vertical axis represents the dimension of "tension" (or, if you like, potential for energy transformation within the system). At the bottom are values representing low tension, and at the top are those representing high tension. These two axes form a grid with four equal quadrants. We shall label them:

1. Left bottom: hypofunction, low tension. (The Chinese would call this *Yin* in *Yin*.)

2. Left top: hypofunction, high tension. (*Yin* in *Yang*.)

3. Right top: hyperfunction, high tension. (*Yang* in *Yang*.)

4. Right bottom: hyperfunction, low tension (*Yang* in *Yin*.)

Simple changes in activity ("function" axis) correspond to the GAS stage/mode 1 ("alarm"), unless they are prolonged. Prolonged

---

89 Chappell D. *The Unitary Concept of Health*. Silica Publications; 1994. ISBN 0 9524265 0 1.

changes in function lead to changes in "tension": this is the GAS stage/mode 2 ("resistance"). The lowest values on the "tension" axis represent stage/mode 3 ("exhaustion"), of which the left bottom quadrant is the most advanced phase.

Archetypal Paths to Ill Health

I propose that the evolution of disease draws a path across this grid, and that the paths it draws may be described in a limited number of stereotypical ways.

The primary deviation from the norm is a tendency towards greater or lesser activity. If normal physiology is plotted as an area in centre of our grid, these changes are represented by shifts to the right or left respectively. If such changes are prolonged, then the baseline or basal tone of the variable will shift (allostatic adaptation). After this, various things may happen.

Paths Departing from Heightened Activity

There is hyperfunction, that is, a response is produced at a lower threshold stimulus. With regard to the SNS, this will translate as resource utilisation for goal-oriented or defensive behaviour. Psychologically it will manifest as nervousness, aggression, fear, hostility, or impatience. Energetically the system will become "highly strung", with high potential for energy transformation or discharge. What happens next depends on the underlying vitality of the individual. So long as the high energy state can be sustained, there will be gradually increasing stiffness (decreasing elasticity). Our plotted point, now to the right of the grid, will shift upwards. The PNS up-regulates to offset the imbalance caused by high SNS activity. But SNS and PNS will interact less precisely, and visceral function will become irregular, with spasms and changes in motility and secretion. Eventually, the organism will no longer be able to sustain the high energy state, and will yield to exhaustion. Our plotted point will slowly sink to the lower portion of the grid as the organism loses vitality.

Paths Departing from Reduced Activity

Alternatively, there is a general hypofunction, a "looseness". Resource utilisation for goal-oriented and defensive behaviour are reduced, in favour of body maintenance and energy conservation functions under parasympathetic influence. Psychologically and energetically the individual shows less activity and vibrancy. The defensive functions of the organism are under-excitable. The response to adverse stimuli is under-stated. The strategic choices are of stability, caution and disinterested observation. These settings predispose towards slowly developing symptoms of reduced circulatory tone (hypotension), reduced catabolic activity (weight gain) and weakened immunity (susceptibility to infections, such as respiratory, genito-urinary). Analogously to what happens with hyperfunction, the availability of the necessary resources and energy to initiate and maintain a secondary, compensatory response, will determine whether from here there is an escalation to the "tense" state of long-term resistance, or a gradual descent towards eventual exhaustion.

Relevance to Acupuncture

Fundamentally, how we get ill depends on (a) our tendency to heightened or reduced activity of the major control systems (CNS, ANS, endocrine, immune), and (b) our innate vitality level. My thesis is that pathogenesis may be described very well by reference to two variables: the activity of a physiological function (say, SNS activity), and the tension in the system. The basic paths to ill health allowed by this description mirror fairly closely those suggested by

Yves Requena's six types of terrain[90].

- Hyperfunction: "Aggressive" type: *Shao Yang*

- Hyperfunction, high tension: "Tense" type: *Tai Yang*

- Hyperfunction, low tension: "Nervous" type: *Jue Yin*

- Hypofunction: "Passive" type: *Tai Yin*

- Hypofunction, high tension: "Tenacious" type: *Yang Ming*

- Hypofunction, low tension: "Lax" type: *Shao Yin*

This model proposes two fundamental attributes of any pathological process, responsiveness to stimuli (excitability), and tension (potential for energy transformation). If we are able to assess these attributes in any individual, this enables us a certain predictive power, for example regarding the kinds of pathological conditions to which they may be susceptible, the prognosis, and their probable responsiveness to treatment. With regard to the latter, as mentioned in Chapter 4, this information can give us guidance on how to needle: depth, needle manipulation, frequency of treatment.

---

90   Requena Y. *Terrains et Pathologie en Acupuncture*. Maloine; 1980.

Index

www.ingramcontent.com/pod-product-compliance
Lightning Source LLC
LaVergne TN
LVHW020334200726
843507LV00012B/2351